HEALTH-WEALTH FOR YOU

HEALTH-WEALTH FOR YOU

11 STEPS TO SAVE BIG & LIVE HEALTHY

DR. JOSH LUKE

Advantage®

Published by Advantage, Charleston, South Carolina.
Member of Advantage Media Group.

ADVANTAGE is a registered trademark, and the Advantage colophon is a trademark of Advantage Media Group, Inc.

Printed in the United States of America.

10 9 8 7 6 5 4 3 2 1

ISBN: 978-1-64225-081-7
LCCN: 2019930254

Cover design by George Stevens.
Layout design by Megan Elger.

This publication is designed to provide accurate and authoritative information in regard to the subject matter covered. It is sold with the understanding that the publisher is not engaged in rendering legal, accounting, or other professional services. If legal advice or other expert assistance is required, the services of a competent professional person should be sought.

Advantage Media Group is proud to be a part of the Tree Neutral® program. Tree Neutral offsets the number of trees consumed in the production and printing of this book by taking proactive steps such as planting trees in direct proportion to the number of trees used to print books. To learn more about Tree Neutral, please visit www.treeneutral.com.

Advantage Media Group is a publisher of business, self-improvement, and professional development books and online learning. We help entrepreneurs, business leaders, and professionals share their Stories, Passion, and Knowledge to help others Learn & Grow. Do you have a manuscript or book idea that you would like us to consider for publishing? Please visit **advantagefamily.com** or call **1.866.775.1696**.

This book is dedicated to my mother and my inspiration,
Victoria Ann Luke.

TABLE OF CONTENTS

FOREWORD

Those of us working in the field of employee benefits all have that moment when we first recognized the fundamental failure of the US healthcare system. For Dr. Josh Luke, it was his first moment out of a job. For me, it was the loss of a close friend. It's the moment we realized something needed to change.

I started Health Rosetta as a way to help organizations of all sizes end the cycle of ever-increasing healthcare costs for their employees. As Dr. Luke related the story in his prior book, *Health-Wealth: 9 Steps to Financial Recovery*, Health Rosetta plans and advisors have cracked the code for affordable and high-performing, employer-provided care.

However, fixing our healthcare system requires involvement from more than employers alone. Fortunately, there are things that every individual can do to decrease healthcare's present dysfunction, and this book is a guide on how to do just that. Containing medical tactics that can help each of us regain control and cut back on our own healthcare costs, *Health-Wealth for You* puts power back in the hands of the people our healthcare system should be serving.

Dr. Luke and I have a shared passion for reducing unnecessary spending by the thousands, empowering people to take responsibility and restoring the American dream by instead investing money saved in education and communities. Between Dr. Luke's first book and Health Rosetta, businesses have the tools to do their part. Now, it's your turn.

Dave Chase
Cofounder, Health Rosetta

WHY NOW IS THE TIME TO TAKE CHARGE OF YOUR HEALTH AND REDUCE THE COST OF YOUR CARE

Why is now the time for you to declare your family's tipping point on healthcare spending? Consider these statistics for starters:

- In 2018 a family of four will pay, on average, $28,166 for healthcare. This is an increase of $1,222 from 2017 costs.[1]

- Over the past ten years, the cost of healthcare has increased an average of $100 a month for a family of four.[1]

- Healthcare is now America's largest and most influential industry, consuming almost one in every five dollars spent.[2]

- Americans pay double for healthcare what those in other developed nations do.[2]

- More than half of American annual healthcare spending, which totals approximately 9 percent of our gross domestic product, provides zero value.[2]

- In the last ten years, approximately 79 percent of the growth in household income has been absorbed by healthcare expenses.[2]

- Three of four chief executive officers report that healthcare costs are their most serious business concern.[2]

- Commercial insurance premiums have grown almost five times over inflation in the past fourteen years.[2]

- Healthcare expenditures outpaced all other annual household income allocations for middle-class families. While the percent change of all other basic family needs decreased, healthcare costs increased by almost 25 percent.[3]

The time for Health-Wealth is now.

---

1   Christopher S. Girod, Susan K. Hart, and Scott A. Weltz, "2018 Milliman Medical Index," Millman.com, May 21, 2018, http://www.milliman.com/mmi/.

2   Brian Klepper, "How Businesses Can Save America from Healthcare," *Employee Benefit News*, June 9, 2014, https://www.benefitnews.com/author/brian-klepper-1143.

3   Anna Louie Sussman, "Burden of Health-Care Costs Moves to the Middle Class," *The Wall Street Journal*, August 25, 2016, https://www.wsj.com/articles/burden-of-health-care-costs-moves-to-the-middle-class-1472166246.

HEALTH-WEALTH FOR YOU

ARE YOU AN EHC? An Engaged Healthcare Consumer? If not, you are costing your family thousands of dollars a year in wasteful healthcare spending. This book was written for individuals and families who are ready to take control of the healthcare-inflation situation that is financially crippling so many.

The cost of healthcare in America will continue to increase. It's a certainty. It's capitalism. Year after year, your family's health insurance carrier continues to increase your expenses—by at least 5 percent annually, on average. And while Americans complain, many feel helpless and trapped, so they just keep their heads in the sand and continue to pay.

There is a direct correlation between hyperinflating healthcare costs and deteriorating wealth among families in America. As a result, Americans have essentially declared war on out-of-control healthcare costs ... finally! While families have been crying out for relief from skyrocketing healthcare costs for years, it wasn't until 2018 when a series of events led by major global employers gained the attention of those responsible, finally forcing them to enter a discussion on controlling costs. Three of these significant corporate announcements all came in early 2018:

1. In January, Apple announced it was partnering with several major health systems to put your personal health record on your phone.

2. Also, in January, Disney cancelled its traditional insurance carrier, partnered with the local health system, and created its own insurance plan.

3. And in early February, Amazon, JP Morgan, and Berkshire Hathaway formed a new entity to re-create health benefits for their own employees.

Also, throughout 2018 Apple, Amazon, and Tesla all opened onsite employee health clinics at headquarters. These are just a few of those well-known employers who took steps to address the largest uncontrollable expense in their business—providing healthcare insurance for employees and their families.

I am prepared to help you identify similar tactics to the ones these corporations have taken to keep healthcare from destroying your family's financial health and shift this pattern of healthcare consuming a larger-than-needed portion of your family budget. Whether it's better understanding your high deductible plan and how to avoid wasteful spending or simply recognizing the value of understanding your DNA and how your body responds to natural remedies, *Health-Wealth's 11 Steps to Save Big & Live Healthy* will help you and your family begin your journey to financial recovery. And finally, we will lay out the 3P formula to becoming an EHC:

Have a Plan based on Preventative Medicine and Personalized Medicine.

HEALTH-WEALTH: PASSION FUELED BY A SHARED EXPERIENCE

I am passionate about educating Americans on how to prevent Health-Wealth loss from destroying the American dream—in

We will lay out the 3P formula to becoming an EHC: Have a Plan based on Preventative Medicine and Personalized Medicine.

large part because I have directly experienced the system's shortcomings and capacity to threaten families' futures. In 2010, after ten years as a hospital CEO, when a new owner took control of the hospital, I found myself out of a job and my family without health insurance. It was during this same period that my mother was diagnosed with Alzheimer's. I was suddenly thrust into the role of caregiver for my mom while trying to make ends meet for a family that was one medical disaster away from financial ruin, faced daily with the stark, emotional realities of the other side of a healthcare industry of which I was once a part. My mother's diagnosis at age sixty-five with Alzheimer's disease was one of two major events that shaped my life that year. The other, arriving as I was serving my fifth year in the role of hospital CEO, came when President Obama passed his landmark healthcare legislation, commonly known as Obamacare.

Yet it wasn't until almost five years later that the irony of those two events happening in the same year struck me. On January 6 of 2015, I leaned that my mother, who taught me to read as a toddler, was no longer able to read herself as a result of her progressing

Alzheimer's disease. I was angry. I was sad. And I was filled with conviction.

In the same moment I learned that my mother had lost her ability to read, I was overcome with guilt. I had lost sight of the very reason I entered healthcare fifteen years earlier. Poor communication and a lack of focus on patients' needs brought me to a career in healthcare. And now, fifteen years later, I was overwhelmed by the realization that I was now part of the problem. I was a healthcare leader in a broken system, focused solely on capitalism and not on the patients we were committed to serve. I was as guilty of being motivated by "following the dollar" as every other hospital, doctor, and provider. The patient was no longer my priority; I had become part of the machine that is the American healthcare-delivery system.

Health-Wealth is more than just a rhyme. It is personal—for me and for you. In recent years, these two words have represented the antithesis of each other in America. The experiences of watching my mother as Alzheimer's claimed her, and of seeing my own financial future imperiled when I had to choose between my family retaining health insurance or hoping we escaped injury, accident, or disease, are why Health-Wealth is personal to me. I have lived it. I see American businesses closing and families going broke as a result of an industry out of control. If I was not able to afford healthcare for six months after earning a six-figure income for more than seven years, then what percentage of Americans could?

Well, choose no longer. Take control.

HOW TO READ AND APPLY HEALTH-WEALTH FOR YOU

The idea of penning books to teach Americans to save on healthcare spending by pulling the curtain back on the well-kept secrets of the healthcare trade was not originally mine. It was representatives from ForbesBooks who saw my posts online as a social media influencer and subsequently reached out to me and said, "American businesses are hungry for someone to teach them how to drastically reduce spending on healthcare, and we think you are the guy to write the book!"

As a result, this book is the second in the Health-Wealth Series, volumes written specifically to teach Americans how to control healthcare spending while maintaining access to high-quality care and providers. The first book, *Health-Wealth: Is Healthcare Bankrupting Your Business? 9 Steps to Financial Recovery*, was written for American business owners and leaders. This new book, by contrast, is written for you, the healthcare consumer, to teach steps that can save you thousands of dollars. It is a book for the individual, the significant other, the spouse, the parent, or grandparent. The truth of the matter is that the point of both books is the same: individuals must become EHC's if we are to control healthcare costs—we all must engage in the process.

Becoming an EHC is the key ingredient in the Health-Wealth formula.

The intent of this book is not solely to place blame, but to break down the current healthcare delivery model and illustrate how it affects you and your family. The book will provide enhanced knowledge of current policies and their likely impact on you. Those families that recognize the Health-Wealth crisis bankrupting America and are first to adapt to new, specialized programs available to them will reap the financial benefits. This book is your handbook to end the hyperinflation and discover alternative approaches to improve your health and reduce your spending. The result of you reading and acting on the advice of this book will be a healthier you and a happier family as a result of savings of more than 30 percent annually on overall healthcare spending.

> *The result of you reading and acting on the advice of this book will be a healthier you and a happier family as a result of savings of more than 30 percent annually on overall healthcare spending.*

Part I of this book describes the evolution of the American healthcare delivery model in order to establish a basic understanding of why the delivery system is broken beyond repair and why, as a result, costs will continue to increase. This is the old adage of you need to know where you've been to know where you are going. Most of us simply don't have much of an understanding about how health insurance and healthcare work. Many of the most convoluted parts of these systems are that way on purpose, to keep healthcare consumers, confused, uninformed, and overwhelmed. The healthcare delivery model is complicated by design. It is an attempt to disguise the tomfoolery that enabled constant hyperinflation passed onto consumers and corporations over recent years. This was emphatically true in the 1980s and 1990s with the fee-for-service system that was the primary healthcare model. We still live with vestiges of and reactions to this system that long dominated how we paid for healthcare. The real purpose of this book is to help you learn ways to better manage your own care and your own finances, and in order to do that you need to know a little of the history about how we've arrived in the healthcare mess than continues its threat to bankrupt your family.

Part II of the book describes the growth of the consumer-driven healthcare model more commonly known as *high-deductible plans*, and how this model will continue to expand, as it has proven to be effective in increasing individual engagement in critical and expensive healthcare decisions. A better understanding of this current, commonly used insurance mechanism is important to your ability to manage your own care and to make the best family health-care financial decisions.

Part III of the book explains eleven simple, turnkey tactics that you and your family can implement to save more than 30 percent annually on total healthcare spending. These Steps to Save Big will come into play as you develop your Personal Health Plan (PHP), which will focus on improved access, improved health, and reduced spending on healthcare. Section three will teach you how and why bringing the 3P formula to life can save you thousands and improve your health. The 3Ps to becoming an EHC: Have a Plan based on Preventative Medicine and Personalized Medicine.

It's time to declare that your family has reached its tipping point. Commit yourself to leading yourself and your family to improved health and significant wealth. Your Health-Wealth journey begins here.

PART I

HEALTHCARE IN AMERICA: WHERE CAPITALISM WENT WRONG

CHAPTER I

THE AFFORDABILITY CRISIS

IN EARLY 2011, I was serving as a hospital chief executive officer in Southern California. I had accepted my first hospital CEO job at age thirty-two, and had later moved to lead this larger, competing hospital. I had hit my career stride and was on a roll. Then, abruptly, as I mentioned in the prologue, after seven years serving as CEO, the hospital's ownership group made significant staffing cuts, including sweeping leadership changes. I found myself out of work.

After six months of job-seeking, I received two job offers on the same day. My wife and I, after consulting with our children, made the decision to leave California to manage a hospital in Las Vegas. We all missed Southern California desperately and were anxious to move back. Once my employer caught wind that I was actively looking to return to Southern California, they abruptly ended my employment. With my first experience of unemployment I had been provided a severance package that covered our healthcare benefits.

But this time I was forced to decide whether or not to purchase health insurance for my family through COBRA, a 1985 federal legislative act that mandates coverage extension, providing employees the ability to continue health insurance coverage after leaving employment. COBRA offers an opportunity to remain insured—but the premiums can be astronomical.

With the move back to California and without a job, our finances were tight. And when the COBRA invoice came, the monthly premium was in excess of $1,300 and could potentially be as high as $2,000 a month. Even though we had three children under the age of twelve at the time, this expense was hardly justifiable, even for our most precious assets—our children. We investigated other options, and even the most basic benefit packages carried minimum monthly premiums in excess of $1,100—all while unemployed.

So, my wife and I made one of the most difficult decisions of our lives: we decided to live without health insurance for ourselves and our children. It pains me to this day even thinking back on that decision. It was my own personal affordability crisis. I had been a hospital CEO for almost eight years, with a great salary, yet my family could not afford basic healthcare insurance. That's the moment I realized the American delivery system was broken beyond repair.

> *I had been a hospital CEO for almost eight years, with a great salary, yet my family could not afford basic healthcare insurance. That's the moment I realized the American delivery system was broken beyond repair.*

The reason others like us continue to face this affordability crisis is capitalism. Everyone is trying to make a buck. And it's not about Obama or Trump, or a Democratic or Republican majority in Washington, DC. It is about finding an affordable model that meets everyone's needs—a seemingly impossible task.

The cost of raising a family in America will continue to increase. There is no doubt. Inflation, unions, cost of living, interest-rate fluctuations, real estate costs all drive the seemingly uncontrollable costs of healthcare coverage.

In most companies, the most significant year-over-year expense increase in recent years has been the cost of providing health coverage to employees. The annual increases insurers require of American companies, whether mom-and-pop or Fortune 500, have been staggering. In fact, hundreds of companies have gone out of business in recent years simply because they did not foresee how healthcare insurance costs were bankrupting their company. The writing was on the wall and had been for years, but they ignored it—a healthcare version of *The Big Short*. *The Big Short* is a 2015 film that documented how, from 2005–2007, almost every industry and every individual in America chose to keep their heads in the sand and ignore the inevitable as subprime lending statistics demonstrated that a nationally devastating crash of the entire financial and real estate sectors was not only probable but inevitable. In 2007–2008, the United States experienced this crisis, which proved financially catastrophic to many businesses and bankrupted many families.

> *In most companies, the most significant year-over-year expense increase in recent years has been the cost of providing health coverage to employees.*

If only life had a rewind button. The next economic crisis and bankruptcy scare could be yours. If you lost your job or your company struggled, you could be faced with that critical moment when you are forced to decide between paying $2,000 a month or more for family COBRA benefits or taking your chances and going without health insurance. Are you prepared?

So, let me be the first to ask you: *What are you going to do about it?* The future success of your family is on your shoulders. Ever-increasing healthcare costs will bankrupt you if you allow it. Time is running out.

> *Ever-increasing healthcare costs will bankrupt you if you allow it. Time is running out. America's affordability crisis is your family's affordability crisis.*

America's affordability crisis is your family's affordability crisis. It's an American financial epidemic. It's no fault of yours that you have inexplicably been forced to pay huge increases in recent years for health coverage, all while the insurer reduced the benefits afforded to you.

In the hospital business, we have what we call "core staffing." This term simply refers to the bare minimum staff hospitals are legally required to have on hand at all times to care for patients. Hospitals go out of business when revenues no longer exceed the costs of core staffing on a consistent basis. That's capitalism 101.

So, what is your family's "core staffing"? What's that bare minimum of resources required to pay rent and feed your family each month? At what point does your family have to downsize, move to a less desirable town, or run out of funds for basic needs like clothing and food? That's your core staffing.

HOW FEE-FOR-SERVICE BANKRUPTED MEDICARE

In September 2017, FierceHealthcare reported that the costs to employers to provide health insurance to its employees increased for a sixth straight year.[4] Well, that's why I am writing this book. That cost to your employer, entirely or in part, inevitably gets passed on to you. You've seen it; every year your take-home pay decreases, even if you get a modest cost of living increase. Each year you slide backwards a step. Yet you are one of the lucky ones who still have time to study the issue of the inexplicable annual increase in healthcare costs and reverse the trend for your family. The revolution begins today.

"Forget Taxes, Warren Buffett Says. The Real Problem Is Health Care," was a *New York Times* headline after the shareholders' meeting for Berkshire Hathaway in May 2017. Famed American financial icon and company CEO Warren Buffet stated that, about fifty years earlier, "health care was 5 percent of G.D.P., and now it's about 17 percent." Buffet went on to state that "medical costs are the tapeworm of American economic competitiveness."[5] That tapeworm that eats at corporate profits typically is paid for by passing costs along to you, the employee. In essence, your own "G.D.P." continues to fall.

Buffet's response arrived in 2018 when his company announced it was teaming with Amazon and JP Morgan to essentially recreate how healthcare is delivered to American corporations. Buffet, who as of this writing is pioneering this movement with two other powerhouse companies, could ultimately prove to be taking the most significant step to impacting and reversing healthcare hyperinflation

---

4   Paige Minemyer, "Premiums for employer-sponsored insurance increased slightly for sixth straight year," FierceHealthcare, September 20, 2017, https://www.fiercehealthcare.com/aca/premiums-for-employer-sponsored-insurance-increase-slightly-for-sixth-straight-year.

5   Andrew Ross Sorkin, "Forget Taxes, Warren Buffett Says. The Real Problem Is Health Care," *The New York Times*, May 8, 2017, https://www.nytimes.com/2017/05/08/business/dealbook/09dealbook-sorkin-warren-buffett.html.

in America in coming years. Will he succeed? If he does, will it lower costs to you or just save the companies money? Time will tell.

But how did we get here?

In the 1980s, the fee-for-service (FFS) approach and a standardized fee schedule were created to pay doctors for each of the different services they provided, both in hospitals and in their offices. So, other than office visits, if a physician wanted to increase his or her income, patients had to be sick and institutionalized in hospitals, nursing homes, or other post-acute institutions.

So, what exactly is "fee-for-service"? I like the definition I found on Wikipedia in December 2017: "FFS is a payment model where services are unbundled and paid for separately." FFS had been the dominant physician payment method in the United States throughout the 1980s and 1990s, and some elements of it still exist today despite reforms to regulate it. In healthcare, it gives an incentive for physicians to provide more treatments, because compensation is dependent on the quantity of care rather than the quality of care. Fee for service will likely be completely phased out by 2022 as we transition to new models. Similarly, when patients are shielded from paying a higher portion of the overall costs (cost sharing) of their health insurance, they are incentivized to welcome any medical service that might do some good. Thus, some of these "just to be safe" tests and treatments, ordered when insurance shoulders the majority of the costs, would be refused by the patient if the patient was responsible for the additional costs or a significant portion thereof.

I have a shorter, simpler answer for you. FFS is exactly what the name says. Your doctor gets paid a fee for providing you a service. Likewise, the hospital is paid a fee for providing you a service. If you are healthy and never need to go to a doctor or hospital for their services, then they don't get paid. Thus, the goal of doctors and hospitals is to put a head in a bed, so they can get paid—and then order as many tests as they can.

There are a number of problems with the FFS approach. The methodology, as described above, undoubtedly incentivizes and results in overutilization of services and delivery of expensive, unnecessary care. The FFS model financially incentivizes doctors to admit patients to hospitals and post-acute facilities and further rewards them financially for keeping patients in facilities for extended lengths of time. This all gets exacerbated by primary care doctors taking care of their fellow physician buddies by referring often unnecessary tests to them as specialists, which allows these specialists to bill for services as well. While this is not the case for all physicians, of course, it is widely accepted and understood that this takes place in hospitals with a significant number of independent physicians who are not affiliated with or compensated by a larger group but rely strictly on the volume of patients seen daily for their income.

If you are healthy and never need to go to a doctor or hospital for their services, then they don't get paid. Thus, the goal of doctors and hospitals is to put a head in a bed, so they can get paid—and then order as many tests as they can.

To be fair, it was not just doctors that were incentivized to institutionalize. Hospitals and post-acute facilities shared the same incentive. The FFS era drove the heads-in-beds strategy. This is also true for other inpatient providers: nursing homes; long-term, acute-care hospitals (LTACH); and acute rehab facilities, for example, have the same reimbursement methodology. The hospital or nursing home only benefits financially when a patient is admitted or receives care. Thus, the incentive is to find a reason—any reason—to admit a patient or to order additional imaging or lab tests to identify potential concerns.

Are you looking forward to the day that you will be admitted to a convalescent home and told you will be living there for the remainder of your life? Most people chuckle when I make that statement. And that's fair. It's a laughable statement. Of course, no one wants to be admitted to a skilled nursing facility (SNF). Perhaps some of our aging physicians should be reminded of this.

When you visit an emergency department, it is fair to assume that you are there to be evaluated by a doctor to see if care, medication, and treatment are necessary. But that assumption does not align with the reality of the business model of the hospital or the physician. Let's be clear about this business model. You are not in the emergency department to be assessed. You are there so the doctor can identify a reason—in fact, any justification at all—to admit you to the hospital. Why? It's capitalism. In the emergency room of American hospitals, you are a potential widget, and the doctors will run tests and order labs until they can identify a justification to convert you to an actual widget or, in more common terms, admit you to the hospital.

The key operational flaw in the FFS delivery model is that there is no required preauthorization for services. The term "managed care" emerged in the 1980s as a means to control this type of laissez-faire behavior by requiring the insurer to preauthorize any services ordered by a doctor or hospital. Without preauthorization, the doctor and provider do not get paid. There are many forms of managed care, but the one constant is a cost-control measure: written preauthorization from the insurer. Without a required preauthorization, the delivery model was lawless, and much abuse took place. Fraud ran rampant in the healthcare sector as greedy hospital owners and physicians took advantage of an environment with no one at the helm. Thus, I have renamed the FFS era "the fee-for-service free-for-all."

In an era with explosive growth in the healthcare space, where there could not possibly have been enough oversight, the FFS era truly became a free-for-all, and it was lucrative for many. The problem was that the federal Medicare fund was disappearing at an alarming, unsustainable rate, and there was little evidence that this increase in spending was resulting in improved health or improved quality of care.

FFS results in overutilization of services and delivery of expensive, unnecessary care. Patients often simply pay a minimal co-pay regardless of the volume of tests, and in turn patients are incentivized to welcome any medical service that might do some good. There are no checks and balances in FFS. A physician's order for care was the ultimate judge and jury; there was no preauthorization required for admission to these levels of care.

The FFS free-for-all was lucrative for all. One program in particular that utilized the FFS reimbursement model was Medicare. Medicare is the federal insurance program for Americans over the age of sixty-five. In recent years, approximately 22 percent of all Medicare patients admitted to an acute hospital are subsequently transferred to an institutionalized level of post-acute care (nursing home, long-term acute care hospital [LTACH], or acute rehab hospital). Although on the surface one would assume a doctor would only send a patient from the hospital to another institution as a last resort, that is not always the case. One reason for such a high volume of patients being transferred from hospitals to post-acute institutions instead of being discharged home is that their doctors are incentivized financially to keep them institutionalized.

WHAT FEE-FOR-SERVICE LOOKED LIKE IN ACTION

Think about it. Let's provide a hypothetical example of a sixty-five-year-old male. The man calls his longtime family doctor, and this is what takes place:

Patient calls doctor: "Hey, Doc, I fell a week ago, and my hip is still hurting. Should I come see you or go straight to an orthopedic specialist?"

Family doctor responds: "Come see me first. I will let you know if you need to see a specialist." (This is the first unnecessary step in the process, but now the primary care physician gets to bill the payer.)

Patient visits family doctor at his office. Family doctor examines patient and refers patient to the hospital for labs and imaging tests. Family doctor bills payer for office visit.

Patient goes to hospital for labs and imaging tests. Hospital bills payer for services provided.

Hospital calls family doctor with results. The doctor's fishing expedition (to find any possible issue with the patient) pays off, as he finds some minor swelling and a possible minor hairline fracture in one image, both of which would likely have healed on their own and never been a concern of the patient.

Family doctor refers patient to orthopedic specialist.

Orthopedic specialist says he only has office hours two days a week, so it's best to meet him at the hospital. Orthopedic specialist advises patient to go back to the hospital but to report to the emergency room and advise the nurse that the orthopedic specialist told him to come to the emergency department.

Patient goes to emergency department. Patient reports to the nurse his minor hip discomfort from a week-old injury and that the orthopedic specialist advised him to go to the emergency department. Nurse calls orthopedic specialist, who orders additional X-rays and an MRI but does not have time to come to the hospital until twelve hours later, as he has other priorities. Hospital bills payer for emergency services, MRI, and X-ray.

Nurse calls orthopedic specialist. Nurse advises orthopedic specialist that the images have been returned. Radiology doctor hired by the hospital documents that there is a possible hairline fracture but is unsure. Radiologist bills payer for reading images.

Orthopedic specialist orders the patient admitted to the hospital for observation and requests that the family doctor or assigned hospital primary care doctor perform the initial required history and physical upon admission. Hospital doctor (hospitalist) does history and physical on patient, as the family doctor was unavailable to drive over to the hospital that night. Hospitalist is unable to find any pertinent information about the patient documented in the notes or chart, so hospitalist asks the emergency department nurse why the patient is there. Nurse reports, "He fell a week ago and has discomfort in his hip. There may be a hairline fracture. The orthopedic specialist thinks the patient may need hip surgery and wants to evaluate him as a precaution." The hospitalist, who thinks a different exam may be more effective than those images already taken, orders an additional image done and notices some lab results slightly out of range. The hospitalist then orders a consult by a cardiologist. The hospitalist bills the payer.

Orthopedic specialist finally arrives at the hospital. Orthopedic specialist examines the patient, who has been at the hospital for ten hours now, and does not see any need to keep the patient hospitalized any longer. He advises the patient to take Motrin but wants to hold off on discharging the patient until the cardiologist completes his consult. Orthopedic specialist bills the payer.

Cardiologist completes the consult and finds no reason for concern, and discharges the patient home after twelve hours in the hospital. The cardiologist and the hospital bill for services.

All because the patient had a sore hip and needed Motrin. Which either doctor could have diagnosed without running any tests just by feeling the affected area and doing some motion and stretch assessments. Do you wonder now why the Medicare fund is running dry and insurers require preauthorization for services? What if the patient had simply gone to the orthopedic specialist's office first? The result would have been identical, as each of those tests was unnecessary. This practice still continues today (2018).

I gave you a hypothetical circumstance, but it is not at all removed from reality and parallels countless numbers of patients I have met. You, or someone you know well, has likely experienced something very similar. In our hypothetical case, our patient's experience would have created Medicare billings totaling in the thousands of dollars.

The Patient Protection and Affordable Care Act (PPACA), also known as Obamacare, had a triple aim: improved care, better health, and lower cost (efficiency). President Obama's goal to reduce costs may have ultimately come to fruition, had Obamacare survived. But that savings was not going to manifest in this decade, even if Hillary

Clinton had been elected and Obamacare survived. Why? There were too many iterations, innovations, transitions, transformations, implementations, technological mandates, and leadership changes to get it all right so quickly.

So, whether it's under Obamacare or some version of the Trump administration's tweaks to the delivery model, healthcare costs were destined to continue to increase for businesses and families either way after the 2016 election. But what gives? When do American businesses and families reach a Health-Wealth tipping point where they can no longer allow health insurers to increase rates annually for the same or fewer services? Well, that may be up to you.

At current pricing and income levels, it is expected that the millennial generation in the United States will spend more than 50 percent of their lifetime earnings on healthcare. In his book *Catastrophic Care,* David Goldhill breaks down a scenario where the actual percentage may be even significantly higher than 50 percent.[6] This is not practical. In fact, it's frightening. The circumstances I shared at the beginning of this chapter, like the hypothetical example I provided, are only worsening for the generation now entering the workforce.

America's healthcare delivery system is a capitalist's dream, an unstoppable machine with excessive margins at all levels. So long as American businesses and families are willing to pay, the system will continue to spiral out of control. I got into this business to serve senior citizens and make a difference in people's lives. But it became apparent within a few short years that my mission was at odds with the delivery model, as capitalism had interfered long before I arrived on the scene.

---

6   David Goldhill, *Catastrophic Care: How American Health Care Killed My Father—and How We Can Fix It (New York: Knopf, 2013).*

The hurtful truth was this: as a hospital executive, I was now as much a part of the problem as anyone else working in healthcare. I had been labeled an up-and-comer in the hospital space with the skill set to continue this culture of greed for years to come. As a hospital CEO, balancing corporate greed without compromising patient care became more and more difficult with each year that passed.

This culture of greed has bankrupted and torn apart thousands of American families. It will unfortunately continue to destroy many more in coming years. Will your family be the next victim of this culture of greed? The answer may be up to you.

CHAPTER 2

A CULTURE OF GREED

IN 2O14 I WAS ASKED TO SERVE as CEO of an inner-city hospital in Los Angeles. As CEO, I would "round the hospital floors" daily, greeting staff, patients, and guests. I recall walking into a patient room on the medical-surgical unit one morning only to be approached by two middle-aged men. Their body language and facial expressions exuded frustration as I reached my hand out to introduce myself.

"Does our mother have to go to this other hospital the doctor keeps mentioning?" one of the brothers asked, as their aging mother edged to the side of her hospital bed to stand up.

"And how come the doctor is making me stay two more days when I told him I was fine, and the nurse said I was cleared to go, as well?" the patient asked.

Although it would have been appropriate to discharge the patient that day, the doctor had other plans: plans rooted in greed.

By keeping the patient in the hospital two more days, even if she did not need to be hospitalized, the doctor would make an additional $110. And instead of discharging her to recover and heal at home, the doctor was documenting that the patient could benefit from a long-term acute care hospital (LTACH) stay. The average length of stay in an LTACH is twenty-five days, and the referring doctor is reimbursed daily. So, whether she needed it or not, their mom was going to be institutionalized for another twenty-seven days, all for the sole reason that the doctor viewed her as a widget that produced income for him.

I encouraged the two brothers and the patient to chat with the doctor and advised them that they were free to disagree with the doctor at any time and go home.

Medicare reimburses doctors fifty-five dollars a day on average for a routine hospital visit. Medicare guidelines have a baseline length of stay for each patient diagnosis. Patients with their mom's diagnosis had a mean length of stay of five days, even though she had only been in the hospital three days so far.

The doctor was also being paid a monthly stipend by multiple LTACH hospitals and nursing homes to serve as their medical director. While the medical director has a list of monthly responsibilities, for the most part the nursing home or LTACH could live without them. The reality is that these agreements are in place so that the facility can pay approximately $2,500–$5,000 a month to the doctor and in turn benefit from the revenue generated by the doctor sending the bulk of his or her patients to that facility. Thus, there was even more incentive for the doctor to prioritize his own interest well above that of the patient.

Now imagine if this were *your mother who was being told she could not go home for almost a month.*

WILL YOU ALLOW HEALTHCARE TO BANKRUPT YOUR AMERICAN DREAM?

Capitalism. It's everywhere you look in healthcare, and it's bankrupting America, destroying the American dream—your American dream. Your family is the victim of healthcare's villains of greed. This chapter will detail the role each of these villains plays in making healthcare unaffordable and therefore inaccessible for many Americans— even middle-class, working Americans. The corporate villains passing these expenses on to your family include hospitals, insurers, insurance brokers, pharmaceutical companies, device manufacturers, and electronic medical record (EMR) companies, among others.

> *Capitalism. It's everywhere you look in healthcare, and it's bankrupting America, destroying the American dream— your American dream.*

As already illustrated in the prior story, doctors in particular are incentivized to overprescribe and institutionalize. The FFS model incentivizes doctors to admit patients to hospitals and post-acute facilities and further rewards them for keeping patients in facilities for extended lengths of time. There are a number of problems with the FFS approach. The methodology, as described previously, undoubtedly incentivizes and results in overutilization of services and delivery of expensive, unnecessary care—the heads-in-beds strategy discussed earlier. Hospitals and post-acute facilities shared the same incentive.

There is one other component of FFS that completely changed how the doctor approached inpatient care. FFS reimburses a doctor for consulting a patient every day in an acute hospital, an LTACH, or an acute rehabilitation hospital. The more patients a doctor transfers from the acute hospital to an LTACH or inpatient rehabilitation facility (IRF), the more personal income that physician can earn. Once doctors figured out they could bill for services daily in each of these settings, their tactics changed, and they started finding opportunities to justify additional patients going to each of these settings where they could can bill for services daily. It was prevalent during the fee-for-service era and led to significant wasteful spending of Medicare dollars. Welcome to the world of the "quota-based physician."

Quota-based "physicianing" became so entrenched in some doctors' daily routine that it became the norm. They would look for any justification they could to send a patient from the hospital to an LTACH or acute rehabilitation hospital, simply so they could continue to bill for services daily.

So, instead of considering sending the patient home as an option for discharge after being hospitalized, active doctors who focused on caring for senior citizens became entrenched in a culture that they argued was based on "limited physician liability." In the interests of "erring on the side of caution," they would send patients to institutions after the hospital instead of to their homes. "I cannot send these patients home, as I'm liable if they fall and get hurt once they get home," a doctor might say. Those are pretty powerful words. They are certainly words that anyone who is not a physician is slow to challenge. The word *liability* usually ends the conversation, as no one would challenge the physician. It is the same word emergency room doctors use to justify admitting patients to the hospital as opposed to discharging them home from the emergency department—another example of wasted Medicare dollars in the FFS era.

The financial incentive for doctors to practice on a quota basis is significant. Doctors are taught these financially lucrative tactics by the very specialty hospitals that doctors refer patients to. These specialty hospitals, LTACHs, and acute rehab hospitals pay them a monthly stipend for providing allegedly "necessary" physician/advisor quality assurance and support services. Many of these services have been legally challenged as unnecessary. When one of these services contracts expires (usually annually), the service agreement will not likely be renewed if the doctor had not been referring a significant volume of patients to the LTACH or IRF. Guess what? Once those "services" are no longer performed, there is no noticeable impact on the facility, its operations, its quality, or its patient satisfaction. So, I ask you, if the services are "needed" to justify them legally, why is it that when they are no longer performed, no one misses a beat? It is all a sham, that's why.

How lucrative are the financial rewards of employing a quota-based approach for an independently practicing physician? An active doctor who has an average of ten patients a day in legitimate need of the services provided by various acute hospitals would receive reimbursement from Medicare of just under $279,000 annually. However, if that same doctor instituted a quota-based approach and found a justification to transfer as many of those patients as possible to an LTACH or acute rehab, he would receive approximately $672,000 annually in Medicare reimbursement. Sounds like a perfect material for a future episode of American Greed! These costs are passed onto your employer through higher insurance costs and to you and your family through higher premiums.

Quota-based physicians are also notorious for having an acute hospital length of stay that is longer than the norm. The reason they do this is, as always, financially motivated. Even though the patient may be healthy enough to go home after being in the hospital for three days, the physician is often able to collect one to two more days of reimbursement if the patient stays in the hospital. As awful as it sounds, your doctor could leave you in a hospital unnecessarily so he or she can collect an additional fifty-five dollars in reimbursement. Welcome to the FFS American healthcare delivery model.

I operated and consulted for several hospitals where case managers and discharge planners reported examples of overly long hospital stays taking place regularly. It is downright awful. Even worse is that cash-strapped hospitals serving the inner city are often helpless to change the doctor's behavior, even when they have egregious examples. Many acute-care hospitals are so desperate to put heads in beds that they are not about to bite the hand that feeds them by alienating a high-volume-referring physician. It would be career suicide for any hospital CEO to do so. Even though it's an almost inhumane practice, the hospital is helpless in many cases to address it, as the doctor holds the license to practice, not the hospital operator, so we can't overrule them on clinical decisions.

Even in the absence of any justification, the mere fact that physicians are considered experts, along with their ability to document in a way that furthers their own goals instead of documenting the true facts, was enough reason for everyone to look the other way in the FFS era.

As it relates to documentation, physicians can essentially justify anything they desire as long as they have a game plan from the start. Physicians know which tests to order to create a logical path to suggesting someone needs an LTACH visit after the hospital. Even in the absence of any justification, the mere fact that physicians are considered experts, along with their ability to document in a way that furthers their own goals instead of documenting the true facts, was enough reason for everyone to look the other way in the FFS era. I call this "documenting toward the discharge." It runs rampant in hospitals and post-acute facilities, where nurses and administrators often feel helpless to question a doctor's judgement, and it is a means for a doctor to paint a picture suggesting post-acute care is needed by simply knowing which words to write in a chart.

In addition to a lack of transparency on pricing, many leading hospitals are not-for-profit entities, meaning they are exempt from paying taxes. These hospitals are also required to create a community-benefit plan each year to ensure specific community needs are being met. By allowing hospitals to maintain their not-for-profit status, it allows them to become dominant players and reduces the competitive landscape.

For example, if there is a local physician group that sends their high-reimbursement surgeries to a competing hospital, a hypothetical not-for-profit, in many cases, would just go offer to buy the entire physician practice, in turn ensuring that all the surgeries were referred to it. While a for-profit hospital could employ the same approach, there is not a level playing field, as the for-profit is subject to paying a significant amount of taxes each year. While hospitals maintaining not-for-profit status seems to be a hot topic in the media in recent years, there has been little action by individual states to address this issue.

Doctors who are employed or are part of a medical group have less incentive to operate in the capricious manners I have detailed, as they receive a salary in many cases. There are, however, quite a few doctors who prefer to remain independent so that they can practice as individual business owners. As a result, independent-practice doctors have much more incentive to bill as many patients as possible and order as many tests as possible.

Let's think back to chapter 1, where we clarified that emergency room doctors' true intent in the FFS era was not to evaluate you but simply to find a justification—any justification—to admit you to the hospital. The hospital is structured so that it contracts with physician groups for multiple services. Some of these services include emergency department, psychiatric, and others we will discuss later in the book. The point to be made here is that these physicians and physician groups are selected through a competitive bidding process. Ultimately, the hospital will select the group that proves to be the most financially lucrative, meaning the group that is most willing to be as aggressive as possible in putting heads in beds to drive revenue for all.

Just as described with the doctor in the emergency room finding justification to admit as many patients as possible, how do you think the hospital's psychiatrist reacts when the hospitals calls seeking a consultation for a patient who may have a psychiatric need? Let me state the obvious here: the hospital is not calling because the patient does *not* need a consult. Translation: the fact that a primary care doctor or nurse requested a psychiatric consult is traditionally all of the justification a hospital needs to keep a patient hospitalized for days and order a full slate of expensive psychotropic medications for the patient.

Thus, of course, anytime the hospital sees an opportunity to order a psychiatric consult, it is quick to react and encourage the doctor to write the order whether the patient simply suffered confusion, depression, stress, or anything else they could think of, including anxiety. A quick side note here: who doesn't have some anxiety when they are admitted to the hospital? It's a normal human characteristic. I am an advocate for the behavioral health community, a board member for Alzheimer's organizations, and a former CEO of the largest acute psychiatric hospital in Orange County, California. As much as it pains me to share the above information with you, it's the cold-hearted truth of how hospitals maximize revenue. They seek to diagnose psychiatric issues even when they are not present or the reason for the hospital visit. And they are in no way alone. Almost every contracted service in the hospital structure is selected through a competitive bidding process.

The lack of checks and balances for Medicare, which I spoke of earlier, similar to the results of a competitive bidding process, led to the rise of managed care products and ultimately to managed Medicare products like Medicare Advantage. Managed care is the opposite of FFS, as there are checks and balances at every step of the way. As we transition from FFS to managed care, we are currently in a period in which each of these models still exists, but the percentage of individuals covered by FFS will diminish significantly—and potentially be completely eliminated—by about 2023. In fact, these checks and balances must be approved prior to receiving care, even with a physician order. This process is called preauthorization and is common for all health maintenance organization (HMO) product lines. While preferred provider organization (PPO) insurance products often allow the patient to seek primary care without preauthorization, even PPO products in many cases now require a preauthorization for specialized services as well. Both HMO and PPO products routinely offer a "narrow network" of hospitals to clients, which means the insurer and the patient pay less if the patient chooses one of the included hospitals.

But can we pause for a second and ask an obvious question at this point? Why all the middlemen in healthcare? In fact, should we be asking if the insurance company is even necessary? One of the inherent issues with personal healthcare costs is that the health-insurance industry is one of the few industries in the country that has a third party negotiating an individual's costs.

Think about it, you don't have a third party with you at the car dealership when negotiating a car price. You negotiate directly. Negotiation is not just an art that requires intelligence, it is a very emotional process as well. But when necessary, you exercise the ultimate negotiating tactic and walk away when a dealership insists on a price you are not comfortable with. So when will you exercise the ultimate negotiation tactic and simply walk away from your health insurer and demand better?

Have you seen the annual compensation packages of managed care executives and health system executives? They are not poor. Several insurance CEOs take home more than $10 million in one year. I bet that's not the insurer's first message point on the agenda at the annual member town hall meeting! It might be the member's first agenda item, though! Imagine if that $10 million were split up among its members in the form of a rebate check or care credit? That could be a few bucks per member at a minimum. Kaiser Permanente, for example, earned $1 billion in operating gain in the first quarter of 2017. But their average client can barely afford a policy, if at all. And Kaiser is actually one of the more affordable options!

While I am all for capitalism and the free market, at some point, some of these few, very fortunate executives need to get a little closer to reality and understand how that message feels to one of their health plan members who is struggling financially. And this goes for health system executives as well. Everyone is entitled to make a living, and yes, there is great responsibility in these roles, but there are other benefits that can be offered beyond simple compensation that assist in protecting an individual from liability. The federal government should be applauded for attempting to include safeguards in the PPACA to limit the spending and compensation of insurers, but it's a task that was much easier said than done.

Any way you look at it, some of the executive compensation packages in healthcare do not feel good to the struggling single mom or middle-class parents just trying to raise a healthy family. And I can't help but notice that each time I watch a Lakers or Yankees game, the largest advertising banners in the arena and stadium often feature insurance companies or not-for-profit hospitals. While Americans struggle to find the finances to access basic healthcare services, executives from insurers and hospitals are paying six to seven figures a year to wine-and-dine at the ball game in a luxury suite. In fact, at least six health systems nationwide spent more than $1.2 million on television ads alone in 2016, but most of those health systems' clients are likely unable to justify the amount of money spent by consumers on accessing healthcare. So, I ask you, considering our healthcare affordability crisis in America, is this capitalism gone wrong?

Another area of concern that led to America's healthcare affordability crisis involves the compensation packages of insurance brokers cutting deals with businesses. These brokers are often reimbursed on a per-enrollee basis, and their commission is often hidden in the fine print of the deals signed with corporate executives.

We have already discussed several of the obvious culprits in this greed game that led to the affordability crisis, including doctors, hospitals, insurers, and insurance brokers. What about some of the less obvious culprits contributing to America's healthcare affordability crisis, including pharmaceutical companies, device manufacturers, and EMR companies?

Pharmaceutical companies represent another area of skyrocketing prices affecting consumers' ability to afford healthcare. The pharmaceutical industry has always pointed at the Food and Drug Administration's tedious process for bringing a new drug to market as its go-to reason for unjustifiably high pricing. If each new drug patent has a sixteen-year window for exclusivity before other similar generic products can be brought to market, and the approval process takes, on average, eleven years, then the industry battle cry has always been "We can charge whatever we want for the remaining five or six years before generic versions hit the market." While there is truth to this reasoning, the antics and strategies employed by some manufacturers in increasing drug costs in recent years have been well publicized and egregious at times and are a significant contributor to the healthcare affordability crisis in America.

You are well aware of the pharmaceutical company's role in raising your total healthcare costs, but did you know there is actually a middleman between your employer and the drug manufacturer? It's called a pharmacy benefit manager (PBM). The role was originally created in part to serve as an advocate for employers to help them avoid overspending and be more efficient in ordering pharmaceuticals for their employees. Well, it didn't take long for Big Pharma to figure out how to corrupt the PBMs as well. So, although the PBMs were hired to advocate for the employer, their compensation packages have been structured to be more lucrative if they partner with Big Pharma companies.

Where does this affect you? Big Pharma offers cash rebates to PBMs when employees order certain brand-name drugs. Those cash rebates are rarely passed onto the employee or employer but included in the compensation package of the PBM. Further, some PBM agreements prohibit the PBM from even listing any comparable generic medications when a brand name is offered. So, yes, once again you are being suckered by a middleman. These types of programs compromise the PBMs' ability to serve the client with full transparency. After a series of scathing media reports on the lack of transparency between PBMs and the employers they represent, several states proposed legislation in 2018 that requires increased transparency from PBMs as well. Once a popular and valuable resource for managing employee drug spending, many companies, including Coca-Cola, Verizon, and Shell, have already phased out the pharmacy benefit manager role.

Device manufacturers are no exception to this sort of greedy malfeasance. Doctors have a choice of which hardware or device brand to use when operating on a patient or completing a procedure. The margins on many devices are, again, unjustifiable. It's oftentimes just a plastic device, cheap to produce but expensive for the hospital to buy. While hospitals and insurers would prefer that the doctor use the most affordable product, doctors often go with the most expensive version. Why? Whether or not they think a specific product is the most effective, doctors are often compensated by device manufacturers as a means to ensure loyalty. This is very similar to the approach used by nursing homes and LTACHs to contract with doctors as medical directors to ensure referrals. Not surprisingly, this tactic has also been employed by pharmaceutical companies to ensure that doctors write prescriptions for their name-brand products.

Let me give you another example of why healthcare has grown so unaffordable to the average American. There are so many middlemen in healthcare that it is difficult to keep up. These middlemen are all pulling a profit, in most cases at a sizable margin. Look at supplies, for example. While we'd like to think the supply chain is simple and product pricing is straightforward, the supply process may actually look like this:

Manufacturer acquires raw materials	Hard cost
Manufacturer creates product/device	Hard cost
Manufacturer sells wholesale to medical supplier/ distributor	Hard cost
Distributor secures delivery from trucking company	Hard cost
Hospital pays materials management staff to inventory	Salary
Central supply stocks hospital/operating room shelf	Salary
Nurse/physician administer product	Salary
Many devices require a manufacturer's trained rep in the room	Hard cost
Physician bills for application	Insurer billed
Hospital bills insurer for product and application of product	Insurer billed to cover all

Those are the ten steps to get a device to a patient. Each comes with a cost. That cost is ultimately passed on to your employer—and then on to your family.

Electronic Medical Record (EMR) companies are another major contributor to the affordability crisis. Just prior to PPACA a federal economic stimulus package included a series of requirements for hospitals and physicians to implement software and EMR on a short timeline. Do you think that led to lower prices and increased competition? Of course not! It led to price gouging, monopolistic tactics, excessive data blocking, and arrogant, deceptive, and misleading business practices from the leading EMR companies. Why? Because they could. The Feds had their back. And technology is confusing, so anytime the discussion got technical, hospital administrators backed down and trusted the EMR partner and as a result spending grew out of control.

Within a few short months after Obamacare was passed, several big EMR companies were turning away small- and medium-size hospitals as the "account was not big enough to bother with unless you are part of a larger health system." While change may bring opportunity, it did not guarantee innovation or progress in a timely manner when it came to technology, and costs for care shot through the roof as a result, because parts of these expenses were passed onto the consumer by the hospital through price increases. Again, these costs are passed on by hospitals and doctors to businesses and families. All in the name of capitalism!

WHEN CRISIS AND ACCOMPANYING GREED HITS CLOSE TO HOME

All these factors contributing to hyperinflated healthcare costs may seem far-removed from you—until you consider an episode of care that affects you personally. Let me share my own story, by way of example, for it demonstrates so much of what I have discussed.

I lived through an episode with my late grandmother during the last year of her life that exemplified so many of the features contributing to the healthcare affordability crisis. In the summer of 2001, my grandmother Belva's progressing congestive heart failure landed her in the hospital. Both the doctor and the provider (the hospital in this case) were paid for her care during the stay. Rather than ask her if she felt strong enough to go home, as home-based support services were available, the doctor placed his own financial interests ahead of my grandmother's preferences and advised her that she needed to be "transferred" to an LTACH to continue her recovery.

Doctors are very skilled at using terms like "transfer" instead of "discharge," as "discharge" may suggest the patient has a choice in the matter. The truth is, the patient always has a choice in the matter. But for some reason, in America patients are either not aware of that fact or are afraid to speak up.

When my grandmother arrived at the LTACH, she was surprised to learn that she would be staying for more than three weeks. Needless to say, she was disappointed. As was I; she appeared to me to be healthy enough to go home. But remember, both the doctor and the provider get paid at this stop. The "wink-and-nod" between the post-acute provider and the doctor is that monthly stipends are paid to the doctor, and in return, the doctor refers as many patients as possible so that the beds remain full. This clearly clouds the doctor's ability to provide unbiased input to patients in the hospital, as there is significant pressure to keep post-acute beds full.

After three weeks and four days in the LTACH, my grandmother was advised that she needed to continue her care in a "rehab facility." It should be no surprise to anyone that my grandmother stayed exactly twenty-five days, as twenty-five days is the average length of stay required to maximize Medicare reimbursement and maintain licensure for LTACHs. The bigger providers became so good at managing this length of stay within an average range of twenty-four to twenty-six days that *The Wall Street Journal* documented the egregiousness of this financially driven practice, which could not be linked to any sort of improvement in quality of care.[7]

---

7   Christopher Weaver, Anna Wilde Mathews, and Tom McGinty, "Hospital Discharges Rise at Lucrative Times," The Wall Street Journal, Feb 17, 2015, http://www.wsj.com/articles/hospital-discharges-rise-at-lucrative-times-1424230201.

So, after four weeks away from home in two different hospital settings, my grandmother reacted to the news of a "transfer" away from the LTACH by stating, "I thought I was rehabbing here. What is a rehab facility?" The reality is, it's a fancy name for a convalescent home or a nursing home. In fact, the long-term care industry has gone to great lengths in recent years to shed both of those names, replacing them with names such as skilled nursing facility (SNF), short-term rehab, and express rehab facilities. There are two reasons for that:

1. Nursing home reimbursement for short-term therapy days ($300–$700) is two to four times greater per day than the reimbursement operators receive for long-term custodial patients who are unable to live at home any longer ($150–$200).

2. As stated earlier, no one wants to go to a convalescent home (or nursing home). In fact, many years ago, baby boomers promised their parents or grandparents that they would never make the decision to send their parents to a convalescent home. As a result, the industry changed the name in the 1980's to "nursing home" with the hope that patients in the hospital and their family members would not realize their loved one is actually going to a convalescent home (when in fact they are the same thing). Fast forward another generation and now you see the name "nursing home" losing favor for the same reason, and nursing homes are often being referred to as rehab facilities for the same reason! It's industry-calculated changing semantics!

Once she arrived at the convalescent home—I mean, skilled nursing facility—both the doctor and the provider were paid at this stop as well. Now you might be asking, how long does this go on before Grandma Belva gets to go home? Great question. The answer to that question should be the same whether she is in a hospital, doctor's office, LTACH, or SNF. The question is, more precisely, "Is Grandma Belva able to return home safely, and if so, what resources might she require in the home to ensure she will be safe to recover and rehabilitate?" During the FFS era, doctors rarely asked that question, as it would not have been as financially beneficial to them. In fact, each time my grandmother was passed to a different level of care, the financial incentives changed and, in a sense, started all over again for both the new provider and the doctor.

So once Grandma Belva was convinced by her doctor that she needed transfer to an SNF, the very sweet social worker at the SNF advised her that they were hopeful she could heal fast enough to return home after three weeks. Three weeks! Why three weeks? Well, you are getting keen on how the system worked at this point. The longer a patient stays and participates in therapy, the more reimbursement the SNF receives at the lucrative rehab rates. Most patients plateau and no longer show rehab improvement between the tenth and seventeenth day in an SNF. Thus, SNFs try to maximize reimbursement by pacing the patient at a twenty-day rate to lengthen the projected stay and maximize the SNF's reimbursement. By goal-setting for twenty days you can often get the optimal outcome of seventeen to twenty days of therapy.

And let us not forget the two financial incentives for physicians to refer patients to the SNF. They are identical to the two incentives in LTACH: Not only does the doctor get paid again for consulting the patient in a new SNF, but the doctor often collects a monthly stipend ($1,000–$4,000) from the SNF, as well.

Again, this monthly stipend is often part of a sham, a handshake agreement allegedly in place for the doctor to perform "needed services" for the SNF, when in actuality, the understanding is that the doctor will refer a high volume of patients and keep the SNF's beds full.

Finally, after three weeks in the SNF, my grandmother was miraculously ready to return home. However, the doctor advised her that unless she was willing to participate in home health therapy services, she would have to reside in the nursing home for the rest of her life. Wow! What a way to package two options for a senior to choose from. Door number one, please! "I will go home with home health services," she said. And yes, you guessed it, not only does the doctor get a monthly stipend from the home health agency (to refer patients, of course), but the provider and the physician once again billed the insurer.

It's the FFS free-for-all, no doubt about it. And if you were listening very carefully back in Southern California in the summer of 2002, you may have heard a collective cheer from the provider and physician community when my grandmother fell and was rushed back to the emergency room. Yep, it was time to put her back on the forty-five-day merry-go-round and let all the providers and doctors bill for delivering services to her. Imagine a world where providers and physicians actually just met her basic needs and comforted her emotionally, so she could return home safely to age and heal in her own environment. The illustration on the next page shows this service-driven model.

GRANDMA BELVA—CONGESTIVE HEART FAILURE (2002)	
Medicare Dollars Paid to Providers (Does Not Include Doctor)	
Home	$0
Hospital	$48,000
LTACH	$52,000
Nursing home	$12,000
Home with home health	$4,000
Hospital	$36,000
Nursing home	$18,000
Assisted living with home health	$4,000
Hospital	$42,000
Nursing home	$24,000
Hospital	$58,000
Total cost of care	**$298,000**

But since, as we have seen, providers and physicians don't get paid when patients are healthy, patients are often institutionalized unnecessarily for financial gain—whether willfully or not, as was the case with my grandmother. As in a lot of instances, particularly with the elderly, she simply was not made aware of her options and trusted that the doctors were acting in her best interests. But as the above graphic makes clear, her doctors were not taking actions in her medical best interests or basing decisions on what would make her the most comfortable, they abused a rigged system that lined their pockets. In my grandmother's case, her physical needs had reached the point where she was better suited for hospice care than a hospital or nursing home. How did this happen? You guessed it, when doctors order hospice, the unlimited gravy train of billing for services for primary care doctors, specialists, and providers dries up.

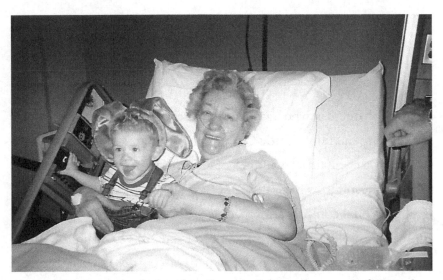

My son Brandon sits on the lap of my Grandma Belva in the summer of 2002 when she was in a nursing home, riding the FFS merry-go-round.

Once a patient is moved into hospice care, a few services can still be provided by doctors, but other than the hospice company and the medical-equipment provider, the unlimited path of unaccountable billing for services for multiple parties ends. In my grandmother's case, it is very likely that home-based services could have been offered and could have improved her care while at the same time saving significant Medicare dollars. And guess what else? My grandmother would have been much happier being cared for in her home. Yet no one ever advised her that home-based care was an option. Why would they—it was not in their best interest.

> *Physicians were partners in the specialty hospital incentivizing experiment—doctors who "shifted to the dark side" in a model that proved to be extremely lucrative for all.*

So, what is the physician's role in this scenario? Physicians were partners in the specialty hospital incentivizing experiment—doctors who "shifted to the dark side" in a model that proved to be extremely lucrative for all. At each of my hospital CEO stops, I observed a handful of doctors who tarnished the reputation of all doctors by abandoning the Hippocratic Oath in favor of capitalistic greed. They shared in the financial windfall of the model just as much as the specialty hospital owners and CEOs, who were pulling in $3–$11 million annual compensation packages at times. And one last point: while technically legal in principle, at the very minimum, what is described in this chapter is not patient-centric and is, in many cases, beyond unethical. Doctors who participate in such unethical behavior have learned what needs to be documented, and therefore abuse is difficult to prevent.

I share this story with you because so many of the factors contributing to the healthcare affordability crisis in America were exemplified by my grandmother's care plan. Quota-based "physicianing" exemplifies a number of the villains we showcased in this chapter, from doctors to multiple providers. Undoubtedly, both she and the Medicare fund paid more than was necessary throughout the process.

Let's be clear here on how these things contributed to the affordability crisis: aside from a few co-payments paid by my family, all of my grandmother's costs for care (much of it unnecessary) were passed on to *you*—to American businesses and taxpayers. When the Medicare fund runs dry, who replenishes the needed dollars? Taxpayers—American businesses—and families.

The handwritten letter my grandmother penned after returning home from the hospital near the end of that episode still resonates with me today. The letter said, "I am anxious to return home next week; four months is a long time to be away from home."

Dear Martine and Josh and Brandon 8-16-01

You have no idea how much it meant to me to have you all come by last night. I am sure the Lord will bless you for taking your precious time to do it.

I am so proud of all three of you - and happy to know how the Spirit of God dwells in your home. You have truly been blessed with such a gorgeous child. He is just beautiful - and his penetrating smile. I can't believe how big he is. He's a little boy - not a baby. I'm sure his baby brother will be just like he is. That shows you what Love can do.

Today it is very hot here and I'm thinking of you at the beach enjoying yourself. I am sure you are having a wonderful time.

→ I'm getting anxious now to get home and get settled. Four months is a long time to be away from home. The longest in my whole life.

Thank you again for coming and taking me out to dinner. It was a great evening.

Love to all
Grandma

XOXOXOXOXO XOXOVOXOXOXOXOXO

With FFS giving way to various managed care models, the likelihood of your aging parents experiencing this type of fragmented care in the future is reduced, but based on the behavior of this small number of doctors who figure out the loopholes in the reimbursement models, it would be wise to stay abreast of the nuances of your health plan to keep an eye out for any continued tomfoolery that may come about that is not patient focused or in the patient's best interest.

CHAPTER 3

A SYSTEM BROKEN BEYOND REPAIR

IN THE FALL OF 2016, my middle son was a freshman in high school and was in the thick of his first year of high school football. One night after bedtime he complained of stomach pain. Because he had just gone through a full-contact high school football season, we were sensitive to any health issues he brought up. We made the decision to take him to the nearby emergency room.

The closest hospital is owned by a nationally known, for-profit chain with a well-publicized, checkered history of transparency. I knew the hospital well, as I had grown up in the area, I had been a patient in the emergency department myself in prior years, and my daughter had been born there. In fact, a few months earlier, their regional medical director contacted me to ask if I would interview for the hospital's vacant CEO position. It was a reputable, local community hospital.

After three hours in the emergency department and a number of tests, they told us that our son was fine. His pain had subsided, and they found no issues. Great, I thought. All's well that ends well.

Three weeks later, several bills arrived in the mail. I was not worried, as my family had a great PPO insurance plan, and this hospital was a contracted provider. I reviewed the bills, and total charges from the hospital alone were $19,908. My responsibility for the hospital component was $3,516. I was even put off at how much my insurance company paid: $7,970. All for three hours in the emergency room and a few tests. And I was also on the hook for the physician component of more than $1,080. The total costs to have my son's stomach ache assessed for less than three hours were almost $4,600.

Maybe they should make this into an ad campaign, I thought. Instead of saying "The wait in our emergency room is less than fifteen minutes!" as is the norm for hospital advertising nationwide, perhaps they should consider saying: "If you have a great PPO insurance policy, come to our emergency room and we only charge you $5,000!" What a deal!

Even having been a hospital CEO, I was not prepared for the surprise and shock I experienced when I opened the invoice. And in this moment, I was asking myself, did we consent to this? Did anyone tell us how expensive it was? I sought justice as a result of a calculated decision by the hospital to avoid transparent pricing. I called and requested a detailed invoice of expenses. A few weeks later, the detailed description of my son's three hours in the emergency room arrived in the mail.

I called the hospital to discuss the bill and request a discount, as I could see that my insurer had already paid them and, based on my knowledge of the actual hard costs that the hospital incurred, I knew that the hospital had likely already covered their costs with the money collected. As a result, my share of the costs was pure profit for them—and a significant one at that! (After reading this book you will have a better understanding of when a discount may be appropriate and how to tactically request one.) The operator advised that they were unwilling to negotiate. I did not send payment and waited four months until collectors started to call. Most hospital companies own their own collection agency. If the collection agency owned by the hospital has difficulty collecting, they then sell each invoice for ten cents on the dollar to an independent collection agency, which then pursues the patient even more aggressively.

While the internal agency would not negotiate with me, in most cases the external agency will. The entire business model of independent collection agencies is to recover their expense plus additional margin. Very few hospitals provide patients with prices in advance of procedures, and most do not make them readily accessible to patients, even when requested.

Want to know how this story ends? As of this writing, it has been more than two years since that hospital visit. In the initial eighteen months my wife and I received two collection calls from the hospital who refused to negotiate and kept threatening to send the bill to collections. It wasn't that we were not willing to pay, just that we were waiting for someone to call who would engage in a rational, logical conversation with us about the costs. That call finally came after twenty-two months. But it was one call, and one adjusted bill in the mail that included a discount stating: "Pay full amount now and its discounted by 15 percent." That was a good start, but they were unwilling to negotiate from there. I wish I had an update to the story. I guess you will have to follow me on LinkedIn to get an update if and when one comes! In any case, this book is meant to empower you to review your bills and feel confident to question charges and request a discount when appropriate, knowing that it will not hurt your credit score either way!

THE MOVEMENT TO VALUE-BASED CARE

Obamacare was designed in large part to end the heads-in-beds mentality. Essentially, almost every care coordination incentive and penalty in Obamacare was implemented to prevent the unnecessary hospitalization and institutionalization so rampant under FFS. In short, the federal government was telling providers, "If you admit someone to a hospital or nursing home who did not need to be there and could have been cared for at a lower level of care, we are not going to pay you, and we are also going to fine you." As a result, doctors would be less and less motivated financially to institutionalize patients as we transitioned away from FFS.

Whether it was the specific approaches of Obamacare or an entirely new model of managed care, now more commonly referred to as value-based care, is here to stay. There is no alternative for the federal government, as the Medicare fund is still on track to be empty in the near future (recent projections show it being empty by 2029) due to the volume of baby boomers retiring daily. FFS and managed care are on two opposite ends of the spectrum. One was a free-for-all, and the other, managed care, has tight restrictions that must be met before rendering care. No wonder hospitals and doctors continue to resist transitioning to managed care. Managed care came with rules and oversight, two things they were unaccustomed to and did not want to deal with. As for the private market, insurers have been all-in with managed, value-based care for years, as it's an effective and lucrative business model.

After former President Obama made healthcare reform his top priority, his goals included making access to healthcare available to all Americans and, at the same time, attempting to restructure the financial model to address the rapidly depleting Medicare fund. The only path to controlling healthcare spending was a conversion to a managed-care model. For Medicare patients, there was already a proven model that had emerged in recent years: Medicare Advantage—a form of managed care for American seniors who qualify for Medicare benefits, which includes checks and balances in the form of preauthorization.. In Medicare Advantage, a senior voluntarily consents to allow an insurance company to "manage" his or her personal Medicare benefit, and in exchange that individual often receives some added benefits, such as dental or vision coverage, which traditional Medicare does not cover. The Medicare Advantage model has proven to be more financially viable for the government, which simply issues a flat amount of money to the insurer on behalf of each patient each month. The insurer is in turn responsible for any care needed (often referred to as *full-risk*).

It's a simple reality to legislators: there will be no money left in the Medicare fund in the near future, and reverting to a model that allows doctors and providers to bill for services at-will is no longer an option.

As a result, America is rapidly becoming a completely managed-care environment for healthcare. This should theoretically rein in healthcare spending—but don't count on it. Free spending and aggressive lobbying by insurers and hospitals are the norm in healthcare, so this conversion will take time. However, the ultimate goal of the new managed-care models is to control spending. Using my son's case as an example, in a managed care environment the hospital and doctors would both be incentivized to minimize tests, charges, and prescribing unnecessary care.

Almost every payer (health plan or insurance company) that has traditionally reimbursed physicians based on how many patients they see each day has now converted to alternative reimbursement methodologies that represent some form of managed care. They started this transition shortly after Obamacare was passed, and for many, it is already complete. For Medicare, however, the aggressive push is taking a lot longer. Doctors and hospitals are dragging their feet every chance they get, as the new model is a threat to their ability to drive volume and resulting income.

In time, however, with the exception of a few lagging and aging physicians who are set in their FFS ways and have yet to retire, behaviors will change, and an entirely new mind-set for physicians and health systems will be in place in coming years. The trend toward managed Medicare will continue.

One of the primary goals of Obamacare was to initiate a national transformation to a patient-centered delivery model. In a patient-centered model, the first question that should be asked by doctors when patients are hospitalized should simply be this: "Can this patient be cared for at home, and if so, what resources are needed to ensure a safe discharge?" This philosophy is at the heart of the "hospital-at-home" methodology. The goal of "hospital at home" is simply to utilize self-management, technology, and resources to treat and care for ailments at home rather than the traditionally required institutionalization.

The biggest challenge during the FFS era, as alluded to in the story of my grandmother, was that no one ever educated her or the family that she had a choice in where to go after her hospital stay.

They also never asked her if she wanted to go to a nursing home at all, or if she preferred to go home.

Remember my grandmother's story when your family member goes to the hospital: That individual has a choice every step of the way. Empower him or her to question the doctor when something is not completely clear. If you take away just a few nuggets from this book, let one of them be this: this is America, and as patients, whether in the FFS era of the past or post-Obamacare which is transitioning FFS into a memory in the next few years, you ultimately have a choice of your provider and what type of care you will be given.

But even with value-based care now entrenched in American healthcare, the biggest flaw in the delivery system remains: anyone on American soil can access healthcare services in any emergency room in the country, at any time.

Yep, that's a fact. To clarify, the hospital or doctor is not legally allowed to ask the patient or family any questions about money or insurance until after the care has been provided. It's the law.

Let me explain. In 1986, the Emergency Medical Treatment and Active Labor Act (EMTALA) was passed, requiring hospitals to provide necessary medical care to any patient who showed up in their emergency room in active labor or with an emergent need. Hospitals are required by law to provide needed care without ever asking if the patient is able to pay until after care is ordered or delivered.

EMTALA, in a sense, guarantees free access to care for anyone in America, including foreigners,

Hospitals are required by law to provide needed care without ever asking if the patient is able to pay until after care is ordered or delivered.

in any emergency room nationwide. Even though the law is specific to individuals in active labor or with an emergent need, the hospital must see the patient to assess if the need is emergent before they can deny them access. Thus, every individual is guaranteed an emergency room consult, whether they are insured or not, for any reason at all. The hospital's liability is significant if they were to turn any patient away without a consult. As a result, most uninsured or low-income families with minimal health benefits often simply use the emergency department whenever needed and do not even have a personal family doctor. As you are likely aware, the cost of operating an emergency department is significant—much higher than the cost of operating a doctor's office—so this trend puts a significant financial strain on the system and contributes to America's affordability crisis. It also results in added financial strain on hospitals in inner-city areas. In summary, the highest cost level of delivery—the emergency room—is the only level of care utilized by many uninsured Americans. Regardless of the reimbursement model, Americans continue to use the emergency room unnecessarily, and ultimately that puts avoidable additional financial pressures on the entire system, and these costs are passed on to insurers and individuals.

The American tax payer—you—is ultimately footing the bill for this expensive use of ERs as health providers for the poor.

During the FFS era, another contributing factor to hospitals seeking to capture additional revenue from paying (insured) patients and overutilizing paying patients when possible (ordering several often-unnecessary labs or tests), was to make up for the lost revenue on those patients who were treated who had no insurance or ability to pay. To summarize, the vulnerabilities in the fee-for-service model that led to draining the Medicare fund at an alarming rate included several key factors:

- Liability. Doctors would rather be safe than sorry. And hey, why not, they all got paid more if they ordered more tests!

- Relationships, nepotism, or quid pro quo. Call it what you want, but doctors adhered (and still do) to the principle of "you scratch my back (financially), and I will scratch yours in return." The more tests that were ordered, the more doctors got involved and billed.

- Justification. Let us not forget the almighty quest for justification, in any way, shape, or form, to admit an emergency department patient to the hospital. Doctors willingly went fishing for at least some medical reason to back it up! Heads in beds, whatever it took.

Fast forward through forty years of creating and implementing these habits, and in 2011, when managed care was mandated by Obamacare, the payer world began to be turned upside down. There were no more widgets to bill for, no more heads-in-beds reimbursement, no more reward for volume. It's a managed-care world now. And all patients, seniors in particular, must be treated as value-based care cases, whether they are or not.

Making this problem even worse is the fact that the current generation of Americans entering healthcare as adults rarely has a long-term personal physician. Remember the days of having a personal family physician? You could call him or her in the middle of the night or walk into the office without an appointment, and the doctor would meet you at the hospital when you were injured or ill. That's no longer the case. The reason? Look no further than value-based care.

As discussed, the term "managed care" emerged in the 1980s as a means to control laissez-faire behavior of doctors and providers by requiring the insurer to preauthorize any services ordered by a doctor or hospital. Managed care is intended to be a service-driven model, and "features" include limited access for patients, restrictions, required preauthorization, and a constant messaging to live a healthy lifestyle.

> *Managed care is intended to be a service-driven model, and "features" include limited access for patients, restrictions, required preauthorization, and a constant messaging to live a healthy lifestyle.*

HOW VALUE-BASED CARE IMPACTS YOU

In regard to managed care contracting, your primary care physician may not contract with any of the insurance plans offered through your business's contracted provider. Americans change jobs often, and the likelihood of an individual taking a new job with a company whose insurance provider does not contract with his or her desired primary care physician is high. And if your insurance provider is an HMO, it's even more likely that your doctor will not contract with your insurer.

There are several reasons why such policies may affect your personal physician. The hospital may no longer allow your primary-care physician to see patients in the hospital. Or, just as likely, your doctor may have chosen to no longer see patients in the hospital for financial reasons. For example, the reimbursement for consulting one patient in the hospital each day may not justify the time it takes the doctor to leave his or her office, drive to the hospital, visit with the patient, document the necessary treatment, and drive back to the office. Financially, the doctor is better off in most cases just remaining in the offices and attempting to consult one patient every ten minutes for six hours of the day to earn his or her desired income.

Doctors' proclivity for in-office consultation is exacerbated because we have entered the age of physician specialization. Many family doctors and primary care physicians are no longer credentialed to care for patients in a hospital setting, let alone a post-acute setting. The financial structure and incentives of the FFS era led doctors to choose their preferred business model. Very few still have an active office practice *and* care for patients in the hospital. In fact, the few doctors who maintain an active office practice and also see patients in hospitals and post-acute facilities almost all have hired partners, nurse practitioners (NPs), or physician's assistants to support them in adequately fulfilling all these obligations.

So, while you may still have a personal family physician, it is likely that your physician would not care for you should you be admitted to the hospital. Who cares for you in the hospital, then? A hospitalist.

To explain the motivation for hospitals converting to hospitalist models, we must reflect back on hospital financial incentives. Medicare reimbursed hospitals on an episode-based methodology during the FFS era. This meant that regardless of how long the patient remained in the hospital, the hospital was being paid a flat rate or lump sum, depending on the patient's diagnosis, severity, and comorbidities. Reimbursement was not at all tied to how long the patient remained in the hospital. Thus, hospitals quickly realized that the shorter length of time that a patient was in the hospital, the more profitable that patient's care would be for the hospital. Managing a patient's "length of stay" became a top priority. Many primary care physicians, who in the 1990s were still caring for their patients when they were hospitalized, had a tough time meeting hospitals' demand to shorten length of stay.

The hospital's financial incentive is to shorten the length of stay to maximize reimbursement, in contradiction to the physician's incentive to extend the length of stay for a few extra days of reimbursement. As a result, the hospital decided to employ or organize doctors into hospitalists groups and compensate them to ensure they were focused on the hospital's financial incentives.

For example, hospital nursing teams conduct rounds each morning with an assigned medical director to review each patient. If, during morning rounds, the care team determines that a patient is ready to be discharged or will be ready by the day's end, the attending physician is notified, as he or she is required to write a discharge order in the chart before the patient is eligible for discharge. For private-practice doctors, if the hospital calls at 10:00 a.m. to advise that a patient is ready and needs a discharge order written, the doctor may not be able to get to the hospital until that night to write the order. This is known as a discharge delay. In some cases, the doctor was not planning to visit the hospital at all that day and would wait until the next morning.

Hospitals quickly realized that they could not rely on these private-practice physicians to reply and write discharge orders in a timely manner. Thus, hospitals began contracting for "hospitalist" services. A hospitalist is a doctor who is contracted with the hospital for the sole purpose of managing patients in that hospital. His or her top priority each day is to identify patients who are ready for discharge and make sure those patients are discharged in a timely manner.

Over time, use of hospitalists became more and more common, to the point that many hospitals converted to an entirely hospitalist model and no longer permitted private-practice physicians to consult patients within the hospital. The hospitalist model is even more prevalent and necessary in managed care than it was in the FFS era, so it is likely to continue being the norm in a post-PPACA environment. In fact, most managed care organizations do not use the hospital's hospitalist group but contract with their own group of hospitalists to ensure that the doctors' incentives are aligned with the managed care organization and not the hospital.

It is ironic when you think about it. Hospitals contracted with hospitalist groups in the FFS era for two very specific reasons:

- First and foremost, they were to admit as many patients as possible to drive as much inpatient revenue as possible to the hospital.

- Then, once a patient is admitted to the hospital, hospitalists were to immediately start planning and developing a care plan to discharge the patient as soon as possible to maximize the reimbursement.

That's it. "Get 'em in and then get 'em out!" That was the secret to running a hospital in the FFS era, and the team of hospitalists in each hospital was responsible for fulfilling this mission. In the new version of managed care, now known as value-based care, the model is flipped on its head and the doctors are paid less for every test they order and every patient they admit.

> *"Get 'em in and then get 'em out!" That was the secret to running a hospital in the FFS era, and the team of hospitalists in each hospital was responsible for fulfilling this mission.*

To take that point even further, physician specialization has evolved; post-acute care doctors have employed a hospitalist model as well to once again ensure that the hospital's financial incentives are the priority. Coincidentally, the skilled nursing facility's financial incentive is to *extend* length of stay, in contradiction to the hospital's desire to shorten it. These contracted post-acute specialists are referred to as "SNFists." In most cases, these contracted SNFists do not have a private practice and do not care for patients in hospitals. They simply spend their entire day *consulting* patients in SNFs and other post-acute facilities.

Remember in chapter 2 when we talked about hospitals having a competitive bidding process for physician services within the hospital, where the winner was whoever could prove they would put the most heads in beds? Hospitalists are actually guiltier of this than any others, including emergency physicians. When the emergency doctor wants to admit a patient to the hospital, he or she must first contact the hospitalist to write the hospital admission order. Capitalism rears its ugly head once again. The emergency department doctor picking up the phone or texting a hospitalist to order a consult is itself all the justification needed for a hospitalist to write an admission order in the FFS era—good formula if you are a hospital CEO!

From a capitalistic perspective, you could summarize the move to the hospitalist model by simply stating that the hospital had to buy the loyalty of the doctor in order to align financial incentives—and not just the emergency room doctors but the attending doctors as well. And that led to the emergence of hospitalists. In a way, it's a "you're either with us or against us" approach to ensure that doctors' incentives are aligned with the hospital's incentives. Whereas a personal family physician is likely to be more receptive and loyal to the requests of the hospitalized patient or his or her family, the hospitalist is very clear on the incentive to admit as many patients as possible and then discharge them as quickly as possible to maximize reimbursement. The patient and his or her family has no prior relationship with the hospitalist, so their input was not a priority. The real priority from the hospital perspective is the bottom line. This is why the days of a personal family physician have gone by the wayside.

The reality is that even in what we refer to as traditional Medicare FFS, in recent years a series of new penalty programs for doctors, hospitals, and other providers who abused the system changed the traditional FFS product to become partially value-based as well. These penalties focus on quality factors, criteria-based decision-making, infection rates, avoidable readmission rates, and referral patterns for post-acute care, among other topics.

So how does this affect you? Well for one, it is capitalism, and change brings added expense. While access expanded as a result of Obamacare, costs skyrocketed for many. It was a prime example of the redistribution of wealth in America. Healthcare costs were not reduced. The taxpayers as a group just offset your personal costs to make care more accessible and affordable for you. But the price of services stayed the same—it was just the government paying for a higher percentage. In fact, in many cases, family health costs reached a Health-Wealth tipping point that led families to opt out of health insurance altogether—myself included for a short time, as discussed previously.

> *Change brings added expense. While access expanded as a result of Obamacare, costs skyrocketed for many. It was a prime example of the redistribution of wealth in America.*

Many providers and physicians are still struggling to see how they will fit in a managed care model, which is completely understandable. This transition has been done in the name of more effective, patient-centered care. The federal government loosely describes *patient-centered care* as an approach that focuses more on the patient and less on how physicians and providers are reimbursed. Another common cliché is "from volume to value." That simply means we are making a shift from a volume-based reimbursement methodology to a value-based methodology that rewards physicians and providers for reducing utilization (testing, appointments, and so on).

Because this change is a threat to the income of both doctors and providers, they have been reluctant to convert to a managed care model. This reluctance by doctors and hospitals, as it threatened their revenue model, is why many of the Obamacare policies were put in place—to force this behavior to change. It became a mandate to convert, but providers and doctors were given several years to make the conversion. Most providers and doctors did little to start the conversion to managed care until just months before the PPACA deadlines began in 2014, as the hospital lobby, as well as the American Medical Association (AMA) physician lobby, is one of the most historically influential lobbies in the country. In short, doctors and hospitals refused to move, hoped for a change of heart through lobbying, and when it did not happen, they scrambled to implement plans to meet minimum requirements dictated by Obamacare in the final months before the deadline. Managed care is a threat to their income; there is no way around it. Welcome to the real-world physician community. It's a world of accountability and required criteria.

Even with Obamacare giving way to GOP tweaks during the Trump administration, the Obama era made access to healthcare a much higher priority in American society as a whole. It is important to note that much of an entire generation, the millennials, have now been raised during their adolescent and teen years in an era in which healthcare for the first time became a right to all Americans. Society, no matter their generation, is rapidly becoming conditioned to accepting healthcare as a right. Equally important, the topic has now been prioritized for years. Just like in business, you cannot giveth and then taketh away. Whether it's a pay raise or added benefit, the American way has always been that once something is given, it can't be taken back. With this in mind, it is important to note that regardless of political affiliation, American public opinion in regard to the access to healthcare has shifted dramatically since 2010.

So, if healthcare is a right to all Americans, and we have freedom of choice to go to whichever doctor or hospital we choose, why won't hospitals disclose their prices for each procedure? They have never been formally asked or required to disclose prices. And because healthcare costs are negotiated on an individual's behalf by a third party, there has never been great demand for transparency in pricing. That trend must end. Employers and insurers must insist that hospitals be more transparent.

To make the problem worse, doctors order a significant volume of unnecessary tests and get paid by the federal government and insurers even when the tests are unjustified. Significant amounts of money are being wasted annually on excessive testing and treatment.

Hospitals are not the only entity lacking transparency in pricing. Pharmaceutical companies, doctors, and device manufacturers are just as guilty. Let me share one example of wasteful spending in the name of capitalism.

The lack of transparency in hospital pricing finally emerged as a conversation in 2017 in at least two states: Colorado saw proposed legislation to delay prices being posted, and the state of California filed a lawsuit against Sutter Health for, among other things, lack of transparency in pricing. Just two of many signs that both American businesses and families had reached their healthcare-affordability tipping point!

This chapter illustrates that regardless of the delivery model, so long as healthcare is free in the emergency department as a result of EMTALA, American businesses, their employees, and the self-insured—in other words, you—will continue to face increased premiums each year to offset those costs. While the FFS free-for-all—where there was no accountability for doctors and hospitals—gives way to managed care, it is likely to slow cost increases; the reduction of pace is not significant enough to prevent annual premium increases being passed along to us all.

PPACA could not solve the affordability crisis, nor will any revised version as long as care remains accessible and free in American emergency rooms. Your family is being burdened with this responsibility. Yet no one is holding the hospital industry or insurers accountable for its outdated and irresponsible practices that have resulted in an affordability crisis in America.

This chapter was also intended to help the reader understand how the delivery system became so fragmented, dysfunctional, and unaffordable to the average American over time. As we progress into the final chapter of part I and move into parts II and III of the book, it will be important for you to understand much of what is discussed in these early chapters to better emphasize the importance of implementing the 11 Steps to Save Big and Live Healthy.

CHAPTER 4

MILLENNIAL CULTURE MEETS HEALTHCARE: KEEPING PATIENTS HEALTHY AND AT HOME

I WALKED INTO 24 HOUR FITNESS for my not-so-regular weekly workout and entered my phone number on a keyboard and then scanned my fingerprint to confirm it was me. Ten seconds later I walked into the gym. Wow, that was simple—modern technology. This process makes me feel like a hip millennial!

Why can't hospitals simplify in this manner?

What if each time someone walked into an emergency room anywhere in America, we had at our fingertips a complete medical record since birth for that patient? What if alongside the electronic medical record (EMR), there was cloud-based software that also allowed input from providers, family members, and caretakers of our conversations, observations, and other things pertaining to the social determinants of healthcare, which are often more relevant than the EMR history itself? What an obvious way to enhance your EHC.

What if it simply took a fingerprint and an identification number to access this complete personal history? Either way, it would move us closer to personalized medicine, instant registration and reduced wait times for patients, and decreased nonproductive time for physicians and hospitals. This is my vision for the future of healthcare. If 24 Hour Fitness can do it, why can't billion-dollar healthcare systems?

> *What if it simply took a fingerprint and an identification number to access this complete personal history?*

With that in mind, other questions arise. Why don't we already have more data about patients? Why don't we know more about patients when they show up in the emergency department? Why is it so difficult for health systems to get connected electronically? With all the software providers and innovations available, shouldn't we be further along in terms of knowing more about an individual's health history than we do?

These are all valid questions. I get asked them a lot. The answer is simple: hospitals have had this technology available to them for years but have chosen not to purchase or implement it. After all, it was not conducive to their "don't ask, don't tell, just admit, then bill" approach to caring for patients in the emergency department.

In the FFS era, hospital operators did not want to know more about patients who were showing up to the emergency department. After all, if hospitals had information to prove a patient was not in fact ill or injured, then the hospital would not have been able to admit them to the inpatient floor of the hospital and bill for the care delivered. Remember, heads in beds was the name of the game. If the hospital knows absolutely nothing about the patient, what a great way to justify admitting the patient and get paid. Without electronic records, this scenario could be repeated over and over again each time the same patient sought treatment.

Why bother to be informed about a patient or learn about his or her real medical needs? This may seem laughable, but this is an accurate example of how our country has operated since the late 1980s. The hospital has always been the power player—the king of the hill. So, in a model where the hospital is paid for putting heads in beds, why would the hospital invest in technology that could hinder its ability to admit patients? During the FFS era, there was little incentive for the hospital to invest in advanced technology and EMRs.

The federal government put an end to that myopic mentality when it passed Obamacare, which included aggressive mandates for hospitals to implement EMR systems. These mandates are referred to as "meaningful use" and were implemented in phases. Hospitals were penalized if they did not adhere to these deadlines. The passing of Obamacare and the implementation of a value-based delivery model put tremendous pressure on health systems to do the right thing for the patient in a myriad of ways.

So now we face an age where we have these gigantic software providers and EMR companies, and they send an army of sales and tech support people into the hospital. And yet, these juggernaut EMR providers have not accomplished even the simplest of tasks that would be in the best interest of the patient. While many health systems are getting closer to the model described in my dream scenario at the beginning of this chapter, the technology had been available for several years, long predating Obamacare, and still the profession has been slow to react. Now with incentives and penalties under effect with Obamacare, the "limit access to information and admit at all cost" model is not viable moving forward.

Making use of the technology is but one hurdle in the larger shift towards ending a "heads-in-beds" philosophy so long entrenched. In 2016, as I consulted with hospital CEOs across the country, several prominent executives confided in me that their most significant operational challenge in transforming to value-based care was getting the support of their own hospital-based doctors and case management staff. And even those executives who felt they had the full support of their case managers were expressing frustration that the journey to taking a "discharge home first" mentality within their hospital was proving to be difficult, if not impossible.

As discussed earlier, the incentives of the FFS free-for-all led to deep-rooted cultural practices and behaviors among doctors. As I have chronicled, the pattern became to discharge patients to institutions such as nursing homes or acute rehab facilities after a hospital stay. Not only did it reduce the liability of the doctor and hospital (should the patient return home and then have a fall or unfortunate incident after being discharged), but it also became the easiest and quickest way to discharge a patient from the hospital, as you did not have to coordinate a pickup with the family or, potentially, for additional resources (equipment or drugs) needed at home. Yes! The path of least resistance became the preference for all involved. So instead of going home after a hospital stay, seniors were routinely discharged from the acute hospital to nursing homes, whether it was necessary or not.

As time went on—three decades in all—doctors got much better at justifying why nursing homes were supposedly a "better and safer" option for patients upon discharge than "taking the risk of going home." Combine that with long-standing Medicare regulations that ensure Americans have a voice in choosing a post-acute facility, and doctors felt empowered to control the process. All the doctor had to do was get the patient to agree with his or her recommendation. It became the accepted norm that institutionalizing patients on discharge from the hospital was the more appropriate path.

Patients and their families were led to feel that, by returning home, they would be unsafe and potentially at risk—in their own home. That's not just manipulative, but also extremely powerful when you look at it from a distance: convincing all patients that they are unsafe and at risk in their own home without considering each patient's unique circumstances, home environment, and support system. It seems pretty cavalier on the surface as well. I always jokingly ask when I say, "Raise your hand if you can't wait for the day that you get to be admitted to a nursing home for the rest of your life!"

> *Patients and their families were led to feel that, by returning home, they would be unsafe and potentially at risk—in their own home.*

Without personal ownership of decision making and cost comparison in healthcare, there will be little change. The common terminology used to describe this issue in the healthcare field is *self-management.*

THE CASE FOR SELF-MANAGEMENT TO GROW YOUR INNER EHC

Without self-management and accountability, there will be no momentum or support to drive change in America's healthcare delivery system. Patients and families must learn that they cannot trust the opinion of just one doctor, hospital employee, or insurance representative; they must learn to ask questions and do research on their own to ensure optimal health and pricing transparency. Without self-management or a caretaker who makes the commitment to learn, decreased community health and lower cost efficiencies in care delivery will continue to plague the industry.

America's healthcare affordability crisis is worse than ever, and without personal accountability and education on health and wellness, the crisis will only get worse. Self-management and wellness are no longer simply luxuries for the wealthy; they are synonymous with living a healthier lifestyle. Remember just a few years ago when the word "wellness" came with connotations of Eastern medicine and a physician office lobby with calming water fountains, harmonious instrumentals, and an aroma reminiscent of a fully bloomed flower garden? Not anymore. Wellness and healthy lifestyles are two of the most common traits of our youngest generations.

> *Self-management and wellness are no longer simply luxuries for the wealthy; they are synonymous with living a healthier lifestyle.*

Many employers have invested in workplace fitness and health incentive programs for employees. These programs offer rewards, similar to credit card points or frequent flier miles, for making healthy decisions such as quitting smoking, increasing exercise or steps daily, reducing body fat ratio, and eating healthier foods. It's important to note that these programs don't necessarily just reward that fitness fanatic who sits in the office next to you at work and carries her own water bottle with her each day (often with some odd-colored concoction that we are told is some type of unique formula that burns body fat mysteriously). These programs reward everyone who shows improvement and it is often the individual that began the program with the worst habits and shows improvement that can benefit the most in the long run—both in life and in rewards points!

Similar to employers emphasizing health and wellness, some universities are taking the same approach by requiring students to wear Fitbits and translating their physical activity into a fitness grade. What a great example of how technology is opening doors for millennials. Another example of this transition to healthy lifestyles are the gyms that are popping up nationwide, catering to the middle-aged and the baby boomer generation. These gyms are often outpatient rehabilitation facilities that also serve as long-term workout facilities for aging adults. Although the insurer often pays for the first few weeks of recovery and rehab in these facilities, the gyms were created so that individuals can pay privately to continue coming even when they are back to full health (a "24 Hour Fitness" for seniors). One example of this is in Southern California. Dr. Sheldon Zinberg, founder of Caremore, created the concept of Nifty-After-Fifty, a gym designed specifically for seniors. The concept has been so successful that other medical groups and insurers have joined together to invest in these facilities.

These gyms have equipment not only for physician-guided health but also have computers that test and stimulate mental and cognitive growth. Many of these facilities also have dietitians, occupational therapists, nurses, physical therapists, and other skilled healthcare workers on-site for a few hours every week to provide access and support to members.

It's a genius idea when you think about it: the medical insurer, who is financially responsible for your health, is creating an environment that you pay for privately and separately to improve your health. It becomes a desired social routine for many, as well as an integral part of their lifestyle. It's a senior center for active seniors— just don't tell the individuals working out there that they are seniors!

On that note, one thing you will learn working in healthcare is that no one thinks they are old or sick. It is human nature. For many years my grandmother could be heard saying, "I am the youngest person living in this retirement community. The rest of them are old." She said that right up till her death in her mid-eighties (bless her heart!). But let's do the math here. She lived in a senior community that required all residents be sixty or older, and she lived there for twenty years. So, while it may have been true that she was one of the younger folks when she moved in, it turns out I was the typical gullible grandchild who, twenty years later, was still believing her when she would take me to the shuffleboard park and tell me she was the youngest resident in the park. Looking back, there was a fat chance of that being true when she was in her eighties!

All this considered, it is likely that insurers will start providing financial incentives to patients who live healthier lifestyles. It is likely that regulations will begin allowing insurers more liberty in returning cash discounts to patients who commit to healthy lifestyles and consent to electronic monitoring to prove it. Sound familiar? It's the same approach that auto insurers have been taking to discount auto rates for years. Healthcare insurers are slower to change, as healthcare is one of the most highly regulated industries in the world, and healthcare finance is no exception to those stringent regulations.

Qualcomm and UnitedHealth announced a program in early 2016 called United Healthcare Motion that gives enrollees in United

Healthcare insurance plans wearable devices that have the ability to track how many steps they take each day. Employees who use the devices can earn up to $1,460 per year in savings, which will be placed in a health savings account (HSA). The transformation to healthier lifestyles supported by corporations (who are paying high premiums for health insurance) has begun!

The majority of the technological advances that bring efficiency to the delivery system require a commitment from the individual. That commitment could be time, effort, investment, or simply learning a technology—think Fitbit, iPad, calorie-counting applications, or simply logging into the individual patient portal that is used by your hospital. These tech-based health advancements enable us to have accountability. This is another way you can control part of your own fate and elevate your EHC. We can't count on others to keep us healthy. Thus, caring for oneself and technology become more critical—an area where millennials clearly have the advantage! While millennials no doubt feel picked on at times, they are more prepared for the incoming trends in healthcare delivery, which are rooted in technology and self-management.

LEARNING FROM MILLENNIALS

Let me ask you a question: If you were in your mid-twenties and were told that 40 percent of your lifetime income would have to be allocated for your personal healthcare expenses, would you be all right with it? Or would you say, "What if I live healthier, can

"What if I live healthier, can we reduce that cost?" It's amazing what we can learn from millennial behavior, is it not?

we reduce that cost?" It's amazing what we can learn from millennial behavior, is it not?

Millennials have been raised in an era where self-management of one's personal health has been entrenched in the fabric of their upbringing. Since PPACA was passed in 2010, a sizable percentage of millennials will have little recollection of an era in which FFS was the model, diet and fitness were not a priority, and technology wasn't available at your fingertips 24/7 to assist individuals in making better decisions that affect personal health. The cost of healthcare and paying for insurance is most often not a relevant topic until individuals graduate college and pay for it themselves! All they know is the post-PPACA mentality. Now, it would be naïve to assume that the culture that will result from the drastic changes mandated by the PPACA is complete. Millennials are just young enough that the key cultural trends that emerge—the instant use of healthy technology and the importance of self-responsibility and management of one's health—are likely to be a core component of millennial thinking for their entire lives. As a result, a healthier and more responsible society will evolve, and it is likely that these same individuals will see a rapid rise to leadership positions in the healthcare space.

Unlike Gen Xers like myself who have displayed a pattern of unhealthy issues, such as poor dietary choices and a lack of activity that led to problems associated with obesity, millennials benefit from technology that enables healthy decisions that are readily available, affordable, and accessible to everyone. As a result, it has become much easier to make healthy decisions. Thus, dietary habits are improving, and fitness is becoming more of a priority.

There is a strong likelihood that Gen Xers had just enough exposure to the FFS era that we are too jaded to fully understand and pioneer the necessary change to a value-based, patient-centered model. Think about it. The two models are in direct contrast to each other, and experienced healthcare executives fought the required change that was mandated by the PPACA out of basic human nature, if nothing else. Everyone resists change, but when the change is a complete threat to everything you have ever been taught in your professional career? Yikes!

It's my belief that many healthcare organizations will skip over Generation X executives when looking for their leader of the future and look directly to a millennial who grew up knowing only technology, patient-centered care, and how to succeed in a value-based model. No bones in their body will resist the change! An inherent excitement exists for being part of the transformation to a more humane model—patient-centered care. Should we consider the same approach in your home? Could your family benefit from the approach millennials have taken?

This chapter illustrates how physicians and seasoned executives in healthcare have turned their heads from technology for years, as it was contrary to their revenue model. The material partnered with other sections that showcased how financial incentives, bad habits, and the path of least resistance led to overutilization of healthcare services and resources, as well as institutionalizing patients in hospitals and nursing homes unnecessarily. As the emphasis shifts to self-management, personal engagement, and healthy lifestyles, the common traits of the millennial generation are in line to drive these initiatives in your workplace. This combination of recognition of bad habits and necessary cultural changes can lead to improved health and significant savings for your family.

With this in mind, Part I of this book explained the American healthcare affordability crisis and why the system is broken beyond repair. With this baseline understanding of the motivations and flaws in the current delivery system, you are now prepared to discover, in Parts II and III, the importance of consumer-driven healthcare, a Health-Wealth corporate culture, and eleven tactics that could save you up to 30 percent annually on your healthcare spending. We wrap up Part I with three questions:

1. Are you prepared to embrace the characteristics associated with millennial culture that improve health and reduce healthcare spending?

2. Are you prepared to infuse a culture of self-accountability, self-management, and living a healthy lifestyle into your home?

3. Are you ready to declare, on behalf of your family, that you have reached the Health-Wealth tipping point?

PART II

OWNERSHIP OF HEALTHCARE DECISIONS AND SPENDING

YOUR EMPLOYER NOTIFYING YOU of your annual premium increase has become as certain as the Internal Revenue Service calling upon you each April. The time has come to fight back.

This book was written for individuals and families who are ready to take control of the healthcare inflation situation. Did you know that current estimates show that at least 40 percent of a millennials' lifetime earnings in America will go to healthcare? If your carrier continues to increase your rates more than 5 percent a year, your company may not even survive long enough to see what percentage of a Gen Zer's income will have to go toward healthcare costs!

Part II of this book provides an explanation of how important consumer-driven healthcare and establishing a Health-Wealth culture have become. Beyond housing or rent, healthcare costs are likely your family's second, third, or fourth largest expense. Yet to date, your family has been helpless to manage these increased costs. *It stops now.* Today you begin your journey to become an EHC. You will be provided the tools and insight to develop your EHC strategy—a plan based on personalized and preventative medicine. Reduced wasteful healthcare spending and a healthier lifestyle await!

> *Today you begin your journey to become an EHC. You will be provided the tools and insight to develop your EHC strategy—a plan based on personalized and preventative medicine.*

CHAPTER 5

AMERICANS MUST BECOME EHC'S— ENGAGED HEALTHCARE CONSUMERS

IMAGINE CAR SHOPPING FOR YOUR DAUGHTER. Your daughter did all the research at home and decided on the exact car she wanted, down to every specific detail. Then, you head downtown with your daughter, full of excitement, seeking the best deal you can find on a safe new car for the most cherished aspect of your life. When you arrive on Auto Plaza Drive, you discover that the car you are looking for is offered by multiple dealerships. There are two new car lots, one on each side of the street, each with a different owner. The exact car you decided on is offered on each lot, down to the very last detail—the same name brand, same color, and the same upgrades on both lots.

There is only one difference: the price. On the left side of the street, the car is listed at $16,000. On the right side of the street, it's listed at $42,000.

Why would anyone pay for the $42,000 car when they knew they could save more than 50 percent? The answer is that they might buy from the more expensive lot if they were paying with someone else's money and had no skin in the game.

When consumers spend other people's money without consequence, they are more likely to consider opting for the more expensive option—even if the products are identical—than they would be if it were their own money. That's just human nature. It's the same game in healthcare.

Welcome to the world of American healthcare! Individuals who are free to choose providers without any financial consequence will do exactly that. But in truth, it's not without consequence!

For example, when an individual is having an elective procedure and is asked to choose a provider, the two closest hospitals might fit the following description: Hospital A is reputable hospital twelve miles from the employee's home, and Hospital B is a reputable hospital one mile from home. The employee is asked to make a decision that bears no financial consequence to him or his family, as the co-payment is identical at each facility.

There is a difference for the employer covering the patient, however. The price for the procedure at Hospital A is $16,000, while the price for the exact same procedure, often with the same exact doctor, at Hospital B is $42,000.

Similarly, when employees need a specific procedure and have already hit their maximum out-of-pocket benefit, they quit caring what it costs the company, and that cost can have a variance of $20,000 or more. This is why many employers have started charging employees 10 percent of costs above their maximum and doubling the employees' out-of-pocket minimum if they do not use a *center of excellence,* often referred to as an in-network provider by the employer. Also known as *centers of value,* these are simply high-quality hospitals and doctors who are willing to share prices and lower rates to form a partnership with the employer and insurer. And guess what? It has worked. Employees are now paying attention. You should be such an employee and be aware of these repercussions.

There are plenty centers of excellence out there. Many are struggling financially, so they are anxious for you to engage their services. These centers are the pillars by which your consumer-driven model is built.

Employers are more frequently referring employees to centers of excellence, specifically for high-cost procedures including: hip replacement, back surgery, fertility, and bariatrics. In 2013, Walmart and several other major employers went so far as to contract with only four hospitals nationwide to serve as centers of excellence to perform free hip and knee replacements. Employees could still choose local providers, but then they would have to pay.[8] In fact, in 2017 almost 50 percent of hip replacement surgeries were performed at centers of value, up from approximately 40 percent in 2016. In November 2018, Walmart announced that the program was no longer voluntary and that employees would now be required to have specific procedures at centers of excellence.

The point here is simple: price matters, and quality care is available at centers of value.

These kinds of decisions by corporations allow their employees to focus on quality of care rather than cost. Similarly, at age sixty-five,

---

8   Ayla Ellison, Beckers Hospital Report, "2017 Study of Large employers (National Business Group on Health Study)," accessed December 3, 2018.

Americans become much less focused on the cost of care, as Medicare used to cover almost all of the costs of care. But as the Medicare fund continues to run dry at an alarming rate, benefits have been trimmed, and the cost of care for seniors is once again becoming more of a priority. If you fall into this age category, part of your education should factor in these changing Medicare circumstances.

The point here is that if you are covered by commercial insurance, you are spending your money without consequence because the employee's financial responsibility may be capped, while the employer's is not. This chapter will discuss tactics to change your mind-set to take a much larger interest in the financial impact of your healthcare-related decisions. This concept is known as *consumer-driven healthcare*. Oftentimes, consumer-driven plans are referred to as *high-deductible plans*. While this is true in some cases, there are significant benefits to the plans as well. What you must come to understand is that when your employer is required to pay more, ultimately in one fashion or another, so will you.

Until the turn of the millennium, most companies offered generous health-insurance plans. Individual employee responsibilities were most often annual deductibles under $500 with 20 percent co-pay. When benefits are this strong, there is little incentive for the employee to be motivated to make educated choices on healthcare. It was initially viewed as simply shifting costs from the employer to the employee but has proven to be so much more. Consumer-driven methodologies can significantly reduce spending on healthcare for both the employer and employee, and overall employee health will improve as well. By the time PPACA passed, more than half of the employers in America were already implementing consumer-driven tactics or policies.

Whether you are completely new to the concept of consumer-driven healthcare or converted to the model in prior years, this book and chapter will have plenty more tactics to consider adding to your arsenal to eliminate wasteful healthcare spending. Your financial well-being depends on it! Each year, additional consumer-driven tactics are identified that encourage individual engagement in healthcare decision-making.

HOSPITAL PRICING TRANSPARENCY (OR LACK THEREOF) DIRECTLY AFFECTS YOUR FAMILY

Have you ever asked yourself why certain hospitals can charge outrageous, unjustifiable prices for the same procedure offered at more than 60 percent less across the street? The frustrating answer is "because they can." The American commercial health insurance model to date was conducive to allowing this laissez-faire approach by those with insurance. This lack of accountability from the individual employee has played a major role in driving up your company's healthcare costs.

Whether you are completely new to the concept of consumer-driven healthcare or converted to the model in prior years, this book and chapter will have plenty more tactics to consider adding to your arsenal to eliminate wasteful healthcare spending.

Most hospitals refuse to post prices and will not even make them available when requested by the patient. And the doctor is even more disconnected and unaware of the hospital prices. That's exactly how the hospital wants it. There is no transparency in hospital pricing.

Likewise, there is no consumer accountability to prevent this behavior, so hospitals continue to raise prices year over year.

One of the hidden secrets of hospitals is that they consistently impose significant annual increases on high-volume procedures and impose smaller increases on lower-volume procedures. Thus, the number of total procedures that have rate hikes each year may be small, but profits increase as a result of the increases impacting the high-volume procedures.

A good test to see if the hospital you are considering is transparent to begin with is by asking them to share their procedure prices in advance. Although it is a federal law, as late as 2018 less than 30 percent of hospitals were proactively sharing their prices. In 2018, federal legislation passed laws implementing financial penalties for hospitals that do not post prices.

Interestingly, there is no evidence to date that a correlation between price and quality exists in healthcare. However, similar to the car business, there is a correlation between volume of procedures done and quality. The more cars a dealership sells, the higher the customer satisfaction. Likewise, the more surgeries a doctor does, the higher the quality. Thus, a key indicator of quality in many cases would be to identify the doctor or provider who completes the highest volume of the specific procedure you are seeking. Surgeries are different than admissions. That's an important distinction. When you need surgery, you pick a good doctor, so you go after one who completes a high volume of procedures. By contrast, you are rarely able to pick which doctor assesses you in an emergency room.

The American Hospital Association (AHA), the hospitals' lobbying body, and the AMA, the physician lobbying body, are two of the most powerful lobbying organizations in the country. The AHA and AMA have long been known for making significant campaign contributions that have, in part, allowed this price gouging of the American public to continue. There has been little legislative pushback on the cost of healthcare, even though corporate and personal insurance rates have doubled at least two to three times since 2000. The national healthcare debate has nothing to do with reducing costs, and as a result there has, to date, been little momentum to force providers to be transparent and publish prices, which would in turn force competition.

The political healthcare debate is simply one of cost shifting and redistribution of wealth. The discussion in Washington is masked as a conversation rooted in affordability, but the topic of controlling hospital prices is not at all part of the conversation. The debate is simply focused on who ultimately will pay for these outrageous hospital prices: the individual who consumes the services or the American taxpayer? It's simply a debate of cost shifting, and it is such a passionate debate that it serves as the perfect distraction for elected officials to avoid being called out on the fact that there is little pressure being put on hospitals to both reduce prices and post them regularly. On the insurance side, while slow to do so, many insurers (including Anthem) publicly post a significant number of prices for procedures and include associated physician fees as well.

The debate is simply focused on who ultimately will pay for these outrageous hospital prices: the individual who consumes the services or the American taxpayer?

Critics suggest consumer-driven healthcare is just a means to shift costs from the employer to the individual. While there may be some truth to that, those individuals who engage are likely to receive higher-quality care and save significant money as a result.

We have yet to discuss the issue of consumer trust when it comes to complying with trusted expert's advice. In healthcare, that expert is one's personal doctor's advice regarding which hospital is ideal for care. Patients' commitment to utilizing the facility their doctor recommends is one of the biggest obstacles in getting individuals to take ownership of the financial component of the provider decision. Doctors are now often employed by a health system or, at minimum, financially incentivized by a system. Thus, doctors almost always refer patients to the system they are affiliated with, regardless of price. In most cases, the doctor has no idea what the cost to the patient and insurer is at each hospital, or the difference in price between two facilities. The expense to the patient and insurer is simply not the priority of the doctor. While many Americans have already ventured toward consumer-driven care, this chapter includes a comprehensive list of tactics that very few have implemented across the board.

ENGAGE! BECOME AN ENGAGED HEALTHCARE CONSUMER

When individuals embrace the consumer-driven approach, the result is a financial win and, more often than not, improved health and patient satisfaction. The goal should be to implement as many of these tactics into your lifestyle on your journey to becoming an engaged healthcare consumer, one who can reduce spending and improve health.

The following are some critical steps to adapt to a consumer-driven model and a detailed list of other tactics to research and consider.

The first step is to complete the *Health-Wealth Personal Loss Assessment*—see the appendix for a partial sample and find the actual assessment at www.Health-Wealth.com. Be conscious of the fact that not all of the tactics listed are a good fit for everyone. In fact, without completing the Health-Wealth Personal Loss Assessment, implementing these tactics can actually be extremely costly to your family and may not provide any savings at all.

Next, empower yourself to respectfully challenge and question care recommendations made by doctors and other clinicians, to solicit specific details on why they are making the recommendation, and to ask what the other options might be. For example, these are some questions you should feel empowered to ask:

- Why this hospital?

- Is that the only test I will need to determine the problem?

- What are my other options?

- What are the risks of not following through?

- Is there a generic drug that might be more cost efficient and equally effective?

- Would I be able to avoid another appointment if I am willing to self-administer or take some preventive steps on my own?

Next, utilize resources that assist you in better managing your own health. For example. LetsGetChecked (www.letsgetchecked.com/us/en/) is a medical technology platform that connects consumers to laboratories with convenient, confidential, and affordable solutions to manage personal health. The company provides more than thirty at-home health tests under four general categories of "Wellness," "Women's Health," "Men's Health," and "Sexual

Health." For example, consumers can self-collect lab samples in the privacy of their home or on the go and mail it back to the lab using a prepaid self-addressed envelope. The company offers support from their medical team twenty-four hours a day as well, regardless of the patient's results or outcomes.

Other beneficial resources to enhance self-management include mobile applications that allow you to manage your personal health, or that of a child or an aging parent in the form of a "group chat" or "group text." But these chat rooms that allow you to add caregivers, doctors, family members, doctors, pharmacists, and more, also are often equipped with instructional videos for applying equipment or self-administering. Two I have been impressed with that have platforms with this capability to assist you in managing your own health or a dependent's are MeUCare (www.meucare.com) and LoopdIn (getloopdin.com) from Shift 3 Technologies (www.Shift3Tech.com) in California.

Additionally, give yourself the encouragement and confidence to challenge the differences in the available options, including hospitals and ancillary providers, such as imaging-services providers and labs, and how their pricing structures differ. Also, investigate the cost of the complete episode of care, not just the procedure (in hospitals there are almost always separate invoices from physicians and ancillary service providers). You can do this by requesting an estimate of all costs in advance. In addition to the hospital's bill, specifically request estimates for all ancillary providers, physicians (such as anesthesiologists, emergency room doctors, or radiologists) and all other providers. A good way to start this conversation with the hospital admissions or pre-registration office is to ask, "Who all can I expect a bill from when we are done here other than just the hospital?"

Even after the hospital stay concludes, when it comes to therapy and rehabilitation, ask at every step of the way, "Do I need a doctor, nurse, or therapist to help me complete this activity, or can it be done on my own?" The savings can often be $100 an hour if you can self-administer. Once you have the confidence to engage at this level, you are on the path to success, as you have begun the journey of taking increased ownership in your personal health decisions!

A key step in engaging in the process is obviously the personal financial commitment. The free healthcare option offered by employers may be more tempting for a majority of individuals (the incentive to choose the high-deductible plan is that there is no annual premium or monthly payroll withheld from the employee) if the monthly individual component exceeds fifty dollars.

Now that we have used the example of the car dealer, let's use a true commercial (employer-provided health insurance) healthcare example (see accompanying chart, as well) with the deductibles and coinsurance from the previous paragraph.

Prior Model

You or a family member are having an elective procedure. Let's assume it's the first procedure of the year and is an elective surgical procedure costing $10,000. Under the pre-consumer-driven plan, there was little motivation for you to engage and shop. The company would have paid $7,500, and your personal employee expenses would be $500 out of pocket and coinsurance of $2,000 (0.20 × $10,000), for **a total cost to you of $2,500.**

New, High-Deductible, Consumer-Driven Model without Employee Engagement

In a consumer-driven model, at the beginning of the year you may have opted for the "high-deductible plan," and now you have the opportunity to research and reap the benefits of doing so. For this exact same procedure, you now have two choices. If you went to your favorite local hospital (Hospital A), the price is still $10,000, so you would pay a $1,000 deductible and $3,000 (0.30 × $10,000) coinsurance payment. So, the total would be $4,000, and then you would exhaust the HSA of $1,000, for **a final out-of-pocket bill of $3,000.** Your employer would pay the balance of $6,000.

New, High-Deductible, Consumer-Driven Model with Employee Engagement

In turn, if the you were given information on competition in the local market and chose a center of excellence offering the same procedure at $4,000 instead of $10,000, the bill would look more like this: a $1,000 deductible and $1,200 (0.30 × $4,000) coinsurance payment. So, the total would be $2,200, and you would exhaust the HSA of $1,000, for **a final out-of-pocket cost to you of $1,200.** This represents a savings of $1,800 for you.

Boom! That's no small potatoes for one procedure! And how many times a year do you or a family member need a procedure?

Here's a well-kept secret. Your employer's cost would also be significantly less, totaling $1,800. That's a savings of $5,700 over the pre-consumer-driven plan, and more than $4,200 was saved by simply choosing the center of excellence.

It's that simple. Your employer wins either way in the new model, as the costs dropped $1,500 even if you do not engage and they save a whopping $5,700 when you do engage by choosing a center of excellence.

	Prior Model	New, High-Deductible, Consumer-Driven Model without Employee Engagement	New, High-Deductible, Consumer-Driven Model with Employee Engagement
Procedure Cost	$10,000 (Hospital A)	$10,000 (Hospital A)	$4,000 (Hospital B)
Employee Out-of-Pocket	$500	$1,000	$1,000
Employee Coinsurance for Procedure	$2,000 (0.20 × $10,000)	$3,000 (0.30 × $10,000)	$1,200 (0.30 × $4,000)
Total Employee Out of Pocket	$2,500	$4,000	$2,200
Employee Health Savings Account	None	$1,000	$1,000
Total Employee Spend	$2,500	$3,000	$1,200
Employee Savings (Loss) Compared to Prior Model	N/A	($500) * Appears to be cost shifting, as employee did not participate in the savings.	$1,800 * Evidence that the new model is NOT cost shifting when employee participates.

This chart assumes the annual employee premium remains the same in each model.

After considering these examples, the question is this: How do we bring informed consumer choice to life? Most industries are required to provide a detailed list of all required services to the consumer in advance of providing the service. Some industries even require consumers to sign an extra form that says they understand what was disclosed to them. Why is it the opposite in healthcare? The provider asks the consumer to prove their ability to pay, yet is unwilling to provide any information about services necessary and associated pricing. It's almost laughable how hospitals have turned the tables on consumers, hidden prices, and used scare tactics to collect outstanding debt.

Often, hospitals tell you the cost of a procedure but do not include the ancillary costs or physician component in that quote. Yet when the invoice arrives in the mail, it's expected to be paid in full. In other industries this would be called a bait-and-switch and would be unethical and often illegal. But not in the hospital industry, where consumers have little recourse to challenge the costs—if the invoice is actually accurate (as invoices are often inflated).

So, I ask again, what are you going to do about this deceitful behavior? In consumer-driven healthcare, individuals must identify these incentives that are strong enough motivate you to become a conscious, engaged healthcare consumer (EHC). The good news here is that in 2018, a federal legislation passed that will penalize hospitals that do not make procedure prices available to the public in advance. Your role in this process is to now request these prices in advance, and the hospital is required to provide them. Don't expect them to post them prominently where it's easy to find them, they are likely to continue the cat and mouse game of forcing you make the request.

CONSUMER-DRIVEN HEALTHCARE TACTICS TO CONSIDER

This is a list, in no specific order, of tactics to consider as you convert to a consumer-driven mind-set:

- Seek out wellness and preventive procedures available to you and your family members.

- Seek a plan that has a no co-pay or a lower cost for a routine doctor's office visit (thirty dollars or less) to keep you incentivized to not go to expensive options such as the emergency room or a twenty-four-hour clinic. Many new plans charge the individual at least $500 for an emergency room visit to discourage unnecessary use.

- Seek a plan that offers no individual co-pay for certain procedures when you choose a center of excellence (as the savings to the employer could be in excess of $20,000!). Beware of not engaging and being subject to much higher, even double the cost to you, co-pay, if you choose NOT to go to a center of excellence.

- Seek a plan that offers second opinions at no cost for elective procedures. For elective procedures, ask your employer to pick up the deductible and coinsurance costs for you when they aggressively shop for a center of excellence and it leads to significant savings for the employer as well.

- Review all of your invoices for billing errors on medical bills. Ask your employer to reimburse you 50 percent of any money refunded by a hospital or insurer for billing errors. Approximately 64 percent of employers offer claims dispute assistance to employees, whether financial or simply providing support.[9] Use it!

These tactics are all about self-management. Until you own the process of managing your own health, don't expect much to change!

There are many tactics to employ in a consumer-driven model, and this chapter by no means represents a complete list. However, once you have completed the assessment and identified which tactics are

---

9   "The Large Employers' Health Care Strategy and Plan Design Survey," National Business Group on Health, accessed November 28, 2017, https://www.businessgrouphealth.org/benchmarking/survey-reports/surveys-of-large-employers/.

likely to have the most significant impact on you, you will have the framework for adapting to, or continuing to evolve into, an EHC.

> *These tactics are all about self-management. Until you own the process of managing your own health, don't expect much to change!*

There is so much more to consumer-driven healthcare that it would be impossible to summarize it in one chapter. You will find elements of a consumer-driven approach and culture in just about every one of the Health-Wealth steps discussed in Part III of this book. The best way to identify which Health-Wealth steps are the best fit for you is by completing the Health-Wealth Personal Loss Assessment. Even if you are already an engaged healthcare consumer, this book will have plenty more offerings to consider adding to your arsenal of tactics to eliminate wasteful healthcare spending. Your family's financial well-being depends on it!

CHAPTER 6

CREATING A HEALTH-WEALTH FAMILY CULTURE

In 2015, I went for a routine physical, and my lab results came back "pre-diabetic." What? I had never had problems like this before. "What does this even mean?" I asked. I went online to get a basic definition of pre-diabetic before calling my doctor to discuss and learned that I needed to improve my diet and exercise more. So, I made some changes and now live a healthier lifestyle. And it was not easy.

If individuals engage and commit to living a healthy lifestyle, it will lead to less healthcare spending and increased wealth for your family. And not just financial wealth—Health-Wealth as well!

As a man of faith and a father, I learned at a young age that you don't identify objectives without assigning them financially measurable outcomes. Employ the same tactic in your family. I employed that same approach in developing the steps, or tactics, for this book.

Instill, as a family value, that living a healthy lifestyle and reducing medical expenditures is a financial asset, no different than owning a home. One family member implementing a personal Health-Wealth plan decreases healthcare spending for the individual and the family!

The goal for your family is to empower and educate each family member to commit to three critical steps that affect your family's Health-Wealth:

- Access personal health information to remain educated on needs.

- Develop a healthy living plan that can be electronically measured daily.

- Stay out of the hospital as much as possible!

When each of your family members is committed to these three priorities, you will achieve a significant Health-Wealth savings.

It's likely that the lifestyle choices of millennials pertaining to diet, activity, and exercise are already healthier than those of their Gen X and baby boomer parents. It is imperative that your family embraces and celebrates these healthy living habits so that they become more infectious.

Further, the millennial generation is accustomed to having technology in their hands at all times. That technology has been entrenched in their lifestyle behaviors as well. This includes fitness apps, dieting apps, Fitbits, and other technology that contributes to their health. As millennials and Gen Z children mature, your family will experience a downward spending trend and improved Health-Wealth because of these kinds of behaviors. Thus, the more aggressive you can be in promoting this culture within your home, the sooner your family will see measurable downward spending on healthcare.

WHEN ALL ELSE FAILS ...

While this book outlines all of the middlemen and "villains of greed" in healthcare who drive up your personal costs, I have found a few heroes in this battle for healthcare afford-ability as well. As this book attempts to educate on how to avoid wasteful healthcare spending, there are times and occasions where we all get stuck with more debt than we can handle in a given month. It's often unforeseen medical bills that cause us to eclipse our monthly budget. There are community resources available to help on some occasions.

One of my favorite new organizations to simplify the process to allow you to save thousands on healthcare is HLTHE.com (https://hlthe.com/). Just as you can donate a percentage of your grocery bill to any charity you designate, HLTHE has created a platform where individuals and corporations can raise money, donate funds, and allocate dollars to be set aside for personal healthcare expenses—your healthcare expenses! Much like a Health Savings Account (as offered by many employees to allow a set amount of your spending on healthcare to be tax free), the platform offered by Hlthe. com utilizes donations to pay for your personal medical bills. How cool is that?!

For example, a company, event, non-profit, or individual can donate funds to the HLTHE.com fund and it is designated as a tax-free donation. The donor can identify individu-als, employees of a company, or patients at a designated hospital as the benefactors of the donation. Then it is up to you to sign up and spend the funds. And it's free to you!

These funds can be used for any qualifying medical expense. If your hospital or doctor is not already a qualified provider, you can assist in getting them approved through a short, simple approval process that Hlthe.com created to streamline the process. I have personally witnessed how programs like this can lessen the burden of a family caring for an aging parent, or the grief of parents sitting in the waiting room of a children's hospital. By taking advantage of that time in the waiting room and assisting a provider through the simple credentialing process (it can often take less than forty-eight hours), by the time you receive the invoice for care you could have that provider approved and funds allocated on your behalf. This process can be done for multiple providers, including but not limited to their doctor, hospital, pharmacy, nursing home, home-care agency, medical supply company, or other healthcare professional. The approval process is simply a means to confirm they have an Internal Revenue Service-issued Employer Identification Number and they are in fact a healthcare provider.

Whether it's a catastrophic accident, an aging parent, a sick child, or just a routine doctor's visit, each of these scenarios is equally appropriate, and you don't have to apply for approval from a third party based on your situation, you just have to make sure funds are donated on your behalf or to a group you belong to.

I am a big fan of simple processes and HLTHE.com fits that model. It is quick and easy and can provide significant financial relief in a timely manner to those in one of the most difficult times of their life.

CONVERTING HIGH UTILIZERS TO HEALTH-WEALTH SUCCESS STORIES

Now that we have discussed programs that all family members can benefit from, let's focus on reducing wasteful spending on our biggest utilizers of healthcare services. The 80/20 rule is a baseline for health costs: historically, less than 20 percent of individuals, predominantly those with chronic conditions, make up more than 80 percent of an employer's overall health costs. As employers become more efficient, that number likely approaches the 90/10 rule, because those with chronic conditions will remain the most difficult to manage. This is likely true for families as well; one individual with a chronic condition can account for the majority of your spending. This is another reason that the steps in this book can be so important in reducing your family's wasteful healthcare spending.

For this reason, it is essential that your family seek out programs designed to manage the lifestyle habits of the individuals responsible for the majority of your family's healthcare dollars. The most common chronic diseases include:

- Coronary disease

- High blood pressure

- Obesity

- Depression

- Asthma

- Diabetes

Up to 20 percent of families have a family member affected by one of these high-cost, chronic diseases. There is much a family can do on the preventive side to more efficiently and cost effectively manage these conditions.

3-4-50 Project

The 3-4-50 project is a program developed just for the purpose of disease prevention. Launched in San Diego County, 3-4-50 focuses on the three activities—tobacco use, exercise, and diet—that lead to four chronic conditions—cardiovascular disease, cancer, chronic lower respiratory disease, and diabetes—that account for more than 50 percent of all deaths.[10]

We know from research and experience that our health behaviors can be influenced by the environments where we live, learn, work, and socialize. Accordingly, community health interventions work best when we are able to create collective impact by providing consistent supports for healthy behaviors across settings.

Why not take a similar approach to managing those lifestyle habits in your life and in your home? By simplifying the major drivers of these four conditions that lead to so many additional health concerns, individuals can live a healthier lifestyle by simply raising their awareness and creating healthy culture environments to avoid temptations such as sweets and tobacco at home, at work, and anywhere else you spend a significant amount of time each week, just as we must discourage a sedentary lifestyle.

With all of these approaches in mind, The Health-Wealth Personal Loss Assessment will provide a good indicator as to whether or not a formal incentive program would be an appropriate fit for any of your family members. If the assessment suggests that you may not initially be a great candidate for a formal program, it will also provide details on steps that will likely move you closer to being ready for a commitment of that magnitude.

---

10   Steve Horan, "The 3-4-50 Framework," Community Health Solutions, 2016, http://chsre-sults.com/3-4-50/.

As we conclude Part II of the book, take the opportunity to stop and challenge yourself with the questions below. Once you have asked and answered these questions, you will be prepared to begin Part III of the book and start putting together your 3P Plan to Becoming an EHC using the 11 Steps to Save Big and Live Healthy.

1. Are you and your family prepared to become EHC's by engaging in the healthcare process?

2. Are you willing to seek out prices for procedures in advance to better understand and save on wasteful healthcare spending?

3. Are you prepared to lead the charge to creating a Health-Wealth culture in your home?

PART III

I I STEPS TO SAVE BIG AND LIVE HEALTHY

A FEW WORDS OF CAUTION before proceeding: It's critical that when you finish reading, you complete the online Health-Wealth Personal Loss Assessment before jumping into any of these tactics. Many of these tactics are very specialized, and the assessment was designed to help steer you directly to those that provide the most opportunity for your family, as well as the provider most likely to ensure success in partnering with your organization. A small portion of the online Health-Wealth Personal Loss Assessment is included at the end of the book, but the complete assessment is available online at Health-Wealth.com/Personal-Loss-Assessment.

ENROLL IN AN ALTERNATIVE INSURANCE MODEL

WHILE MANY OF THE STEPS to Health-Wealth featured in this book are simple, singular concepts, this rule is more about taking a step back and exploring all insurance options available to you. Aside from the traditional, well-known HMO, PPO, and exclusive provider organization (EPO) models offered through major health plans, the launch of the PPACA and employers being permitted to opt out saw the reemergence of some long-standing alternative plans and brought about the birth of some new models as well.

While the futures of specific initiatives introduced by Obamacare are often murky, employers will likely continue to have choices to offer employees when selecting healthcare benefits. Waivers allowing companies of a certain size or less to opt out of the mandate or provide employees with monthly pay "in lieu" of benefits may put those companies in a position to benefit from employees choosing to work directly with a co-op or alternative model, as described below. The growth in popularity of Health Savings Accounts (HSAs) could open up the potential for you to opt out of the company-sponsored plan and choose a faith-based co-op if you believe it will better fit your needs.

This chapter will discuss a few of the more common alternative options that have been growing in popularity in recent years that may be an option for you or your family as a complement to or replacement for your traditional insurance plan. Below are descriptions of three models that have seen significant growth since the passing of the PPACA.

Cost-Sharing Community Model (CSCM)

CSCMs are experiencing rapid growth, as they have proven to reduce costs for individuals and families. CSCMs are designed to increase efficiency by utilizing technology such as mobile application scheduling, immediate virtual or telephonic access to clinicians and physicians for members, telehealth consults, and remote monitoring devices to ensure more efficient care delivery at a lower cost. One key benefit includes being able to choose whichever doctor you prefer—just be sure to confirm the fee structure for cash-pay patients with the doctor in advance.

Healthcare cost-sharing models have existed since the early 1990s and membership for all plans combined was expected to surpass one million by the year of this writing (2018). CSCM combines the consumer-driven incentives of discounted value services with technological advances that allow more timely access and are much less expensive than traditional plans.

One example of a leading CSCM is Sedera Health. Sedera's members present themselves to medical providers as "self-pay patients." Sedera then assists in offsetting medical expenses that exceed $500–$2,500, depending on membership level. Sedera's program can also be paired with additional products such as a MEC plan (minimum essential coverage level for preventive needs), an HSA, or direct primary care. Your Sedera Health member concierge will help with appointment scheduling, physician searches, medical bill negotiation, as well as help members receive discounted surgeries and reduced prescription costs. Sedera Health also partners with Teladoc to provide all members with telehealth, remote-monitoring services, and counseling services. There is no co-pay to access 24/7 services from Teladoc, which serves as an incentive for members to adapt to doing virtual consults. Many members find virtual consults to be extremely convenient, as they can do the consult from the comfort of their home or workplace. An additional benefit for Sedera Health members is access to 2nd.MD which provides timely access to top-tier physicians.

One of President Trump's first healthcare-related moves after being elected was to open the door to the creation of smaller, association-based health plans. This policy loosened several specific requirements included in PPACA allowing for creativity and plans for additional smaller groups, a big win for individuals who did not have access to a corporate health benefit. One of the early success stories in the association field is Fit Health.

Fit Health was designed to target and incentivize members who are committed to the proactive pursuit of health and fitness. Fit Health's mission is to provide a program which helps the sick become well and the well to become fit. The plan offers members the opportunity to protect themselves from the financial burdens associated with large, unexpected medical needs through its partnership with Sedera Health. It also provides members the flexibility to see the medical specialists that they prefer through partnerships with local functional medicine and direct primary care offices. The plan also advocates for proactive fitness and nutrition through partnerships with fitness gyms. The good news is that Fit Health is doing this at a fraction of the cost of traditional healthcare as memberships start at approximately ninety-nine dollars a month.[11]

Faith-Based Cost-Sharing Model

Another form of an alternative cost-sharing model is a faith-based cost-sharing program. Members of a faith-based community pay into the ministry, and monthly fees are applied to other members' medical bills. This is not an insurance product. Members are often required to commit to live the standards of the group or church, including praying for other members, abstaining from sexual immorality, and not using illegal drugs.

Coverage for preexisting conditions is limited, abortions are not covered, and preventive care, routine prescriptions, and mental-health support are not covered expenses in most plans. However, the longer you are a member in good standing, the more goodwill you build up to request that some of these other uncovered expenses be given consideration for coverage.

Monthly dues can range from a low of $125 up to $300 per member, and members are required to pay the first $500 of each health incident before asking the ministry to pay for the balance on covered services. Unlike insurers, most of the ministries are not contracted, so there is no guarantee your bills will get paid. Those willing to par-

---

11   "Functional healthcare which rewards the pursuit of fitness," Fit Health, accessed December 3, 2018, www.sickwellfit.com.

ticipate must trust that the system will be funded when they are in need—there is definitely a "leap of faith" component to it that is not common in the insurance world, where policies are generally assured to be funded and detail exactly what is covered and what is not.

Membership in faith-based cost-sharing plans has exploded since the PPACA became law; individuals belonging to a qualified health-sharing ministry are exempt from paying the fine for not having insurance, as required by the PPACA. According to the Alliance of Health Care Sharing Ministries, more than one million Americans now belong to these organizations, led by membership in Texas and California. There are more than a hundred faith-based cost-sharing ministries nationwide, although many of those are small, individual churches and their congregations. As of mid-2018, most if not all of the faith-based sharing ministries in the United States were Christian.

Faith-based cost-sharing programs offer a less expensive alternative for covering personal health costs, with monthly premiums significantly less than what is required in traditional programs. One of the ways faith-based coalitions are able to keep costs down is that most programs do not cover several preventive procedures commonly covered by traditional insurers. For example, colonoscopies, birth control, and mammograms are not generally covered, and members are left to negotiate a cash price and pay out of pocket.

Most of the faith-based programs ask that the member pay the entire fee for each procedure and then request reimbursement. As a result, members must manage personal cash flow consistently, because they will likely have to wait a few weeks after paying the doctor or hospital before being reimbursed by the co-op. Additionally, state or federal regulators have no influence or control over faith-based programs. As a result, if a member has a grievance or is frustrated by a denial, their options for recourse are limited.

Value-Based Insurance Design (VBID)

Value-based insurance design, commonly known as *VBID*, is exactly what the name describes. VBID models are specialized models incorporating many of the tactics discussed in consumer-driven healthcare. VBID models are based primarily on the tactic of charging patients less for high-value or proven clinical procedures and charging more for procedures and treatments that are considered lower value, with less clinical data to confirm their effectiveness.

The highest-value treatment option is not always the lowest-cost treatment option. If a treatment option is much more clinically effective than a less expensive option, it may still be the higher-value option.

Patients can pay a minimal co-pay or none at all for a procedure determined to be high value, making these procedures more attractive to consumers. Likewise, health plans implement higher cost-sharing responsibilities for patients on procedures and services that have little or no clinical benefit. VBID provides an opportunity for the employer, in partnership with the health plan, to incentivize patients to use high-value, low-cost services with contracted providers. This approach is similar to Walmart's approach to certain surgeries; the costs for specific procedures can vary so significantly from one hospital to the next that Walmart provides the service free to employees when they go to a center of excellence.

According to the not-for-profit consumer healthcare advocacy group Families USA, policymakers and insurers should follow eight guidelines when implementing VBID to ensure that consumers have affordable access to high-value care that is best for them:

- Rely on high-quality clinical evidence.

- Reduce cost sharing for high-value care and, on the contrary, discourage choosing low-value providers by increasing cost sharing.

- Have robust networks of high-value providers.

- Reward providers for delivering healthcare based on clinical evidence.

- Provide resources that clearly explain the value-based benefit structure.

- Have an accessible "exceptions process" to allow consumers to get care that fits their conditions.

- Do not require consumers to participate in wellness programs.

- Regularly evaluate the plan's benefit design and its effect on access to care.

In summary, VBID is a specialized insurance model that employs consumer-driven healthcare tactics to provide choice to patients when selecting procedures and services. The pricing of these services is often based on clinical outcomes, and choosing one provider over the next can prove to be quite costly. As a result of consumer-driven models like VBID, hospitals will be forced to be more transparent and compete for market share and business in a manner that was not necessary in the past. I like how *The New York Times* summarized VBID, saying it will "nudge patients to do the right thing."

The programs discussed under this rule are examples of alternatives to the traditional consumer health plans purchased en masse by employers in America. As Americans look to save money and control hyperinflation of healthcare spending, these alternative models have gained significant traction and proven to be a short-term and long-term path to Health-Wealth.

If you have not done so already, now is the ideal time to set the book down and complete the Personal Loss Assessment at https://www.health-wealth.com/. Once you get to the website simply click on the "Personal Loss Assessment" icon and it will take you just a few minutes to complete. Once complete you will be provided an analysis of your opportunity to save and your projected monthly savings opportunity.

ENGAGE IN INTEGRATIVE AND FUNCTIONAL MEDICINE APPROACHES

THE SECOND STEP TO HEALTH-WEALTH is to implement integrative or functional medicine strategies into your 3P Plan, or your personal health plan (PHP). Why not? Isn't that how medicine was practiced before Big Pharma squashed it? Yes, as a matter of fact, in many ways it was.

I remember first reading about the gluten-free craze around 2010 and being skeptical. Then a good friend mentioned that converting to gluten-free foods was the only thing that has resulted in a noticeable difference in the consistently erratic behavior of his seven-year-old son, who has Down syndrome. But due to his son's inability to communicate in the manner his peers would, it raised my awareness that the observations of his parents and physicians were critical.

Then I met a young lady who was an executive assistant on our senior management team, and one day when she ordered the continental breakfast during our weekly CEO meeting, she mentioned that she had gone gluten-free two years earlier. I kind of chuckled when she said that, and I am pretty sure I offended her. She turned, looked at me sternly, and said, "I was on my deathbed for almost four years, and within days of going gluten-free I started feeling healthier and discontinued my meds within weeks and felt better than I had in years."

While this chapter is not about going gluten-free, it is about considering the root cause of disease and illness instead of always focusing on the effect. The end result can be thousands of dollars in Health-Wealth savings!

Are you aware that most physicians do not receive any training on nutrition in medical school? Does that concern you? It should. Most doctors claim that it's not their responsibility to discuss nutrition with you, that there are other specialists for that. Integrative medicine encompasses the use of a nutritionist to ensure your body is being fed an optimal diet based on your DNA and historical reaction to individual foods and ingredients.

Many people liken integrative medicine to what we commonly refer to as "wellness" in America, which is often associated with Eastern medicine practices. I prefer the term "healthy lifestyles" as opposed to "wellness," as it combines wellness tactics with personal engagement in making wise eating and exercise habits. Integrative medicine addresses the whole person, including mind, body, spirit, emotion, and lifestyle. Some often associate it with naturopathic or holistic medicine. But integrative medicine is actually all those things combined—naturopathic approaches combined with modern, Western medicine practices.

Integrative medicine approaches focus on identifying the root cause of the issue, instead of just focusing on symptoms. One of the primary goals is to prevent additional, often more serious symptoms from occurring. Kyle Hill, formerly CEO of integrative medicine company Harvey, describes integrative medicine in this manner:

> When you combine *Eastern Medicine* philosophies such as nutrition, prevention, and natural self-healing with advanced, evidence-based lab testing of Western medicine, you get a new form of medicine called Integrative Medicine. Integrative doctors view symptoms as warning signs of nutritional deficiencies in the body, environmental toxins, improper body functioning, or unfavorable lifestyle habits. They help patients find the root cause of chronic health conditions and focus on treating the whole person, not just a set of symptoms in perpetuity.

Let's be clear here. There are a lot of people out there claiming to be naturopaths or homeopaths pushing natural approaches who are not physicians and unfortunately end up casting much doubt on the naturopathic medicine approach. These folks are not doctors; they are simply selling a product and trying to make a living. That's not what we are talking about here.

We are referring to medical doctors trained to study the root cause and take a comprehensive approach, not simply write a prescription for a medication that does not always address the problem.

So, let's define integrative medicine: integrative medicine uses natural (unprocessed) health and wellness approaches to address the root cause of disease, often trying to eliminate that root cause instead of simply focusing on treating the symptoms. Integrative approaches complement but do not replace more mainstream remedies, often referred to as "Western medicine" approaches.

Let's also define naturopathic medicine. The American Association of Naturopathic Physicians defines naturopathic medicine as a distinct primary healthcare profession, emphasizing prevention, treatment, and optimal health through the use of therapeutic methods and substances that encourage individuals' inherent self-healing process. The practice of naturopathic medicine includes modern, traditional, scientific, and empirical methods.[12]

Integrative medicine sounds a lot like naturopathic medicine, does it not? Well, it's very similar, but integrative medicine is more comprehensive and combines naturopathic medicine with additional approaches.

Americans' access to sweets, artificially flavored foods, and diet sodas containing scientifically created chemicals that often act as a sweetening replacement for sugar are prime examples of the lifestyle changes in recent years with unknown outcomes—not to mention the growth in popularity of greasy, fatty, and processed foods. These factors have all likely led to an entire new set of diseases and symptoms unfamiliar to prior generations.

The need for expansion of integrative medicine is largely because, in my experience, pharmaceuticals have been largely ineffective in treating many of these newer symptoms and diseases that are becoming more common in American society. I believe there is little evidence that drugs can prevent all chronic diseases but, in most cases, only provide a temporary fix or pain relief.

Most major insurance companies do not cover integrative medicine services, and as a result, integrative medicine consults are not a mainstream benefit offered by most employers. However, for-

---

12 "Definition of Naturopathic Medicine," American Association of Naturopathic Physicians, 2011, http://www.naturopathic.org/content.asp?contentid=59.

ward-thinking employers have started to offer employees integrative medicine consults as an added benefit.

It lacks logic that major insurers have moved away from covering the root cause of disease, but based on my research, when studying the history of integrative medicine, it becomes clear that Big Pharma used its massive budget influence to push integrative medicine into the background in the 1950s. Big Pharma wanted the world to believe that drugs can cure all diseases, and they were successful in establishing that as a core belief globally. Money talks, does it not?

As a result, Americans quit focusing on natural approaches and relied on drugs to make them feel better. Because, in most cases, drugs provide at least a short-term fix, this approach became mainstream, and naturopathic doctors and schools declined significantly in the 1960s and 1970s.

Nowadays, the majority of the top twenty hospitals nationwide have opened up some type of integrative medicine practice. One of the many benefits of integrative medicine is that it is often a cash-pay model, which allows the doctor to spend more time with the patient because the physician's monthly salary is guaranteed in advance (managed-care model) so he or she is not in a rush to invoice as many patients as possible. This increased face time with doctors, whether remotely or in person, is a common theme in several of the eleven Health-Wealth steps. Maybe there is something to it?

As millennials become more influential and economically stable, primary medical practices around the country are implementing integrative approaches and hiring integrative medicine doctors. The millennials demand it. This is how they were raised: to live healthy and take care of their bodies. As a result, there has been explosive growth in the practice of integrative medicine since 2000, after fifty years of it being pushed into the background. Those with chronic diseases often figured out that Big Pharma had no cure or that it was too expensive to access, so they sought alternative approaches.

Integrative medicine supports a movement away from generic drug store vitamins and emphasizes specialized natural approaches. In the case of vitamins and supplements, this means conducting lab tests to see which vitamins and supplements can best meet the needs of your biological makeup. You will learn more about this when we discuss whole genome sequencing. Integrative medicine is an opportunity for families to invest in better understanding each individual family member's body and how to best address each person's specific needs.

Integrative medicine is listed in this book as the second step as it embodies several of the other rules that follow and utilizes several of the other Health-Wealth steps. In a sense, integrative medicine brings many of the recommended steps to Health-Wealth together into one coordinated program.

There are a number of resources that can help you accomplish such coordination, including corporate resources and start-ups. My research on integrative medicine showed that there are a number of companies making a difference in the space, some even offering concierge services. Although tech start-up Harvey entered the market with a bang, they sold in 2018 and have exited the market. Other companies, including Parsley Health and Rezilir Health, have taken comprehensive, integrative medicine approaches, implementing tele-health, remote monitoring, and home-based lab services to ensure a low-cost model for patients. Everlywell, Wellnessfx, insidetracker, and uBiome are among the companies that focus on lab testing, with many offering home-based consultations with functional and integrative doctors, as well as home-based lab testing.

Companies like Ritual.com and TakeCareOf focus specifically on vitamins and natural supplements. There is also a presence of organize food focused players in the market, including ThriveMarket and Brandless. All of these companies focus on natural remedies and fall under the integrative and functional medicine umbrella.

Not all companies in the integrative medicine space are necessarily viewed as integrative medicine providers or supplement suppliers. For example, while you will read more about genetic testing in the next chapter, companies like 23andMe and Helix are more focused on DNA testing and mapping your genetic data. Helix states the following on its website:

> We read your DNA using true next-generation sequencing, which unlocks 100X more data than other companies. Where they do single tests, we assemble, store, and protect your genetic data so you can access and share it with any partner of your choosing without ever having to provide another saliva sample.

Helix offers food, supplements, and wellness products, and each is associated with different gene types and recommended for individuals once they identify their genetic map. Color Genomics, found online at Color.com, boasts that its service helps individuals better understand their risk for hereditary cancers and also focuses on those susceptible to hereditary high cholesterol. Although Helix focuses more on product sales, Color approaches employee health by developing an overall wellness plan to address the findings using multiple treatment plans and approaches. Color has a specific product offering developed specifically to support corporate human resources departments. Another well-known company in the space is uBiome, which claims to be the leading microbial genomics company. Its website states the following:

The human gut is home to trillions of microorganisms, which are collectively known as the microbiome. These microbes play a vital part in our gut health, supporting digestion, and the synthesis of vitamins.

A lot can be learned from the human gut, but that's not what this chapter is about. This chapter is about combining multiple approaches of naturopathic medicine with machine learning and DNA testing. The end result is a road map to healthier food consumption, supplements, and more effective drug regimens based on an individual's genetic makeup. That is comprehensive integrated medicine, and if your company invests in it, it's a direct path to Health-Wealth.

Those active in integrative practices certainly have seen evidence of the value of such approaches. "In my almost twenty years of clinical experience," said Dr. Geoff DePaula, doctor of acupuncture and diplomate in Chinese herbology, "I estimate that I have seen that 80 to 90 percent of all health conditions and diseases can be addressed with a natural, less invasive approach using whole-person natural medicine, which is usually accomplished at a fraction of the cost of traditional medical care." DePaula, who also serves as chief executive officer of IM Health, believes that "outcomes are usually significantly and sustainably better, as this healing approach more often resolves the underlying cause of the condition, and is not just managing symptoms with medication."

In September 2017, another sign of the reemergence of integrative medicine was when the University of California, Irvine received a $200 million donation to launch a new health program to promote integrative medicine. The leaders behind the initiative, Howard Federoff, MD, PhD, and CEO of UC Irvine's health system, and Shaista Malik, MD, the director of UC Irvine's Center for Integrative Medicine, state that other medical schools are too slow to adopt alternative therapies that reveal promise in clinical trials and suggest it is time to transform healthcare to focus on a patient's full range of needs rather than just treating an illness.[13]

So, after learning about a handful of national providers in the space, some very focused on one component of naturopathic and holistic medicine and others providing a more comprehensive approach, it is clear that for individuals who choose to go down the path of integrated medicine, there is significant Health-Wealth opportunity, resulting in improved health and significant savings. Every day new resources for investigating and implementing integrative medical approaches become available. You are wise to educate yourself on this changing terrain of healthcare choices.

---

13   Alia Paavola, "$200M donation to UC Irvine for alternative therapy meets criticism," *Becker's Hospital Report, September 20, 2017, https://www.beckershospitalreview.com/finance/200m-donation-to-uc-irvine-for-alternative-therapy-meets-criticism.html.*

FULL GENOME SEQUENCING AND DNA TESTING

HEALTH WEALTH STEP #3 is to have your DNA test done to identify potential forms of cancer and also better understand how your body metabolizes medicine and food. We will start by offering some background on the impact of this modern approach.

In 2007, Geisinger Health (now named Geisinger), a large integrated health system in Pennsylvania, announced the launch of a pioneering DNA testing and genome sequencing initiative for the local community that would include any Geisinger patient interested in volunteering. This initiative was a bold move, with financial support from the National Institute of Health and several other health organizations. It was a revolutionary launch in 2007, like none other in the United States.

Geisinger agreed to pay for exome (partial genome testing) sequencing for all patients who volunteered to be included in the program. At the time of launch, the goal was simply to build a database to learn from, known as a "biobank," and individual results were kept private and not shared with any patients. Genome sequencing is a personal snapshot of an individual and how susceptible he or she may be to chronic diseases, as well as how to best remedy illness through medication consumption or nutritional consumption. You are likely familiar with the term DNA testing, and genome sequencing is simply a comprehensive DNA test of an individual.

It is as close to personalized medicine as we have come to date. Genome sequencing is essentially a personal road map to improved health that differs from one individual to the next. In recent years, other organizations, including the Department of Veterans Affairs, Kaiser Permanente, Renown Health (Reno, Nevada), and Vanderbilt University, have established similar biobanks that allow them to study the collective data.

Then, in 2013, Geisinger made another bold move by opening up the Geisinger biobank to allow patients to access and learn from their personal information. Geisinger partnered with a pharmaceutical company, which allowed them to greatly reduce the cost of sequencing. The initiative, called MyCode, has already enrolled more than 170,000 patients, 100,000 of whom have already been sequenced, adding approximately 4,000 new members a month. Already, MyCode has identified more than 400 patients with conditions through the program. This is personalized medicine at its finest. It is expected that more than 250,000 individuals will have volunteered and been sequenced by the end of 2018.

"The approach is *population genetics*." explained Dr. David Feinberg, Geisinger's former president and CEO who led the initiative from 2016 through the end of 2018, when we had the chance to speak together at a conference. "What Geisinger is doing—and saying to friends and neighbors, who are also patients—is, 'Would you allow us to look at your whole genome?' With a 90 percent positive response rate, Geisinger exceeded its 160,000th full genome, and anticipates hitting 250,000."

At the time the initiative was announced, the cost per individual for sequencing ranged from approximately $1,000–$6,000 per person. Exome sequencing can now cost as little as $300 per person, and full genome sequencing is currently around $1,000 per person. These costs are for sequencing alone; there are additional costs for analysis.

"Geisinger is one of the only organizations taking a population approach to genomics with our MyCode Community Health Initiative," Feinberg said. "There are definitely some great cancer treatment centers looking at the sub-type of your oncogene and determining medication based on what type of cancer you have. There are definitely tests out there that can look at your genetic profile and determine what medication you should be put on or should be avoided: pharmacogenetics."

Geisinger works with hospital EMR giants Epic and Cerner. As long as the patient has a medical record with a medical record number, they can participate in the program. It is likely that hospitals in your community also work with either Epic or Cerner, as they are the two major players in the hospital EMR space and have significant combined market share. This opens the door to you participating in a similar initiative in your community.

"I think it's great what they are doing at Geisinger. How else can you obtain and utilize a person's biological blueprint, as its written in his or her DNA? And variations in DNA are responsible for the differences in people's appearance, such as having blue eyes versus brown, as well as their physiology, for example being strong versus weak," said Bill Massey, PhD, associate professor at the University of Arkansas for Medical Sciences and clinical assistant professor at the University of Mississippi Medical Center, when we discussed the subject. "There are so many things we can learn, including an individual's predisposition to disease, and their response to particular medical treatments," he said. "Scientists can now read the DNA blueprint of a patient, and based on the known relationships between particular variations in DNA and their impact on biological function, it is possible to predict important aspects of that patient's biology that can be useful in maintaining their health or treating their illnesses."

This start-up cost is the primary reason few companies nationally had ventured down this path. But science and technology have finally progressed to a point that Dr. Feinberg believed that the investment was a no-brainer.

"We're going to prevent heart disease," he went on to say. "I think we can say today that if you're a young woman in central or northeast Pennsylvania, your chances of getting breast cancer are lower than anywhere in the world. Because no one is checking entire populations for BRCA and then acting on it. We are. And by doing so it allows us to treat our patients *before* they get sick and helps prevent life-threatening diseases before they take hold. It's changing the course of their lives and the lives of their entire families."

The Center for Disease Control has created a list of tier 1 conditions, and the MyCode initiative, according to the CDC, alerted more than 268 individuals who possessed at least one of these conditions:

- Hereditary breast and ovarian cancer (early breast, ovarian, prostate, and other cancers)

- Familial hypercholesterolemia (early heart attacks and strokes)

- Lynch syndrome (early colon, uterine, and other cancers)

These are all extremely expensive chronic conditions to treat when a family member starts experiencing symptoms, and many other screening modalities provide limited detection. These conditions are chronic and become long-term liabilities to your financial well-being.

Dr. Feinberg reported that MyCode also identified ninety-one patients at risk for cardiovascular diseases, including arrhythmia, arrhythmogenic right ventricular cardiomyopathy, Marfan syndrome, and heritable thoracic aortic diseases. An additional thirty-five participants were found to be genetically susceptible to various forms of cancer, and seventeen additional subjects were increased risk for other chronic conditions. Again, these are all expensive diseases to treat, so early recognition allows you to begin more efficiently managing and preventing the onset of symptoms.

Hypothetically, assuming your cost for testing was on the high end—let's project $1,000 per family member—if even one family member was found to have a chronic disease or some less-expensive, manageable condition, your return on investment for the test is likely to be less than three months. Now that's return on investment (ROI)! This ROI discussion is hypothetical, but it illustrates the opportunity for improved health and significant Health-Wealth savings.

"So, we have this genetic information, along with clinical information, along with twenty years' worth of electronic health records data for four generations of families. And we're returning results to patients—what is now called precision medicine," Dr. Feinberg added. "But I would say precision medicine is taking care of someone who is already sick. To me, what Geisinger is doing is really *anticipatory* medicine. It's coming up with medically actionable conditions and giving that information back to patients."

Others around the country have ventured into different approaches to DNA testing. The most common area of focus to date has been pharmacogenetics, an emerging science that focuses on each individual's reaction to drugs based on their genetic makeup. Technology has come so far in this area that Medicare began reimbursing for pharmacogenetics-focused DNA testing in 2013.

In a nutshell, a simple cotton swab rubbed on the cheek is sent to the lab and can identify which medications will be effective on an individual and at what dosage. Further, it identifies which medications are not as effective and those that an individual may have an adverse reaction to. Imagine how transformational the results could be if your doctor had a printout of the exact medications your body would react favorably to?

Pharmacogeneticist and neuropharmacologist Dr. Bill Massey is convinced that the opportunity for improved health and savings is significant: "These variations in DNA allow us to understand why one patient may respond to 'Drug X' and another only responds to 'Drug Y,' even though they have the same disease with the same symptoms. The relationship between genetic variations and different responses to specific drugs is the basis for the new science of pharmacogenetics."

Imagine the savings opportunity if you had been taking an expensive medication for years, only to learn that your body was resistant and would more likely react favorably to a much less expensive, generic medication? Or that another family member is actually allergic to a certain expensive medication and that the allergic reaction is the reason an additional medication has been ordered? I could provide example after example.

Knowledge is power, and never is that truer than with genome sequencing.

Nutrigenomics is a scientific discipline focusing on disease treatment through the study of genes and nutrition. Nutrigenomics is at an even earlier stage on the consumer market than pharmaco-genetics, but it can help an individual identify food allergies and potentially harmful antigens in food. Some of the more common findings of DNA testing focused on nutritional consumption are lactose intolerance and gluten intolerance.

Until recently, those suspected of being lactose intolerant or allergic to gluten required a physician visit or blood draw for lab testing. Not anymore. Technology has brought DNA sampling and genome sequencing to the consumer market, and the possibilities of how it might improve individual health seem unlimited.

What's the best engagement you can act on to improve your EHC? Well, for starters see what may already be available to you. For example, Levi Strauss is one company that offers free genetic screenings for its employees to assess their hereditary risks for cancers and high cholesterol. Once offered, more than half of the 1,100 eligible employees took the genetic test. Other companies who have partnered with Color Genomics and invested in genetic testing as an employee benefit include Instacart, Nvidia, OpenTable, Salesforce, Slack, and Snap.[14] Corporations who offer such services to their employees can reduce the cost across the board as they are often offered a corporate rate by test providers. Ask if your company sponsors such testing. If they don't, encourage them to consider doing so.

---

14   Natasha Singer, "Employees Jump at Genetic Testing. Is That a Good Thing?" *The New York Times*, April 15, 2018, https://www.nytimes.com/2018/04/15/technology/genetic-testing-employee-benefit.html.

Applying Genome Sequencing in
Your Personal Health Plan

If your employer does not sponsor free or reduced-cost genetic testing, you should still consider paying for having your genome sequenced and review the results with a genetic counselor. Doing so could lead to improved health and reduce your overall spending on healthcare. This is actually one of the easier and likely most cost-efficient Health-Wealth steps to consider.

If you or a family member is able to identify in advance that you are genetically susceptible to a chronic disease, the ROI from that alone will outweigh the annual cost for your entire family. The savings could be astronomical. Integrating your DNA test results into your plan can be challenging in itself, as your doctor is not likely to have had a significant number of patients request this to date, as this is an emerging trend. As a result, there are several companies that provide user-friendly applications or platforms to assist you in providing your doctor the information in a useful manner.

One example is Pro-GeneX. Pro-GeneX analyzes novel genetic data, delivers results in an easy-to-use digital interface, and aggregates the data. As more people implement this tactic into their 3P Plan, the collection of data will be used for comparative outcomes and ultimately reduce the overall the cost of care for all. The more people who use the technology, the sooner additional data will emerge to better diagnose and recommend remedies for individual patients as well.

Individuals and families should take the bold move of purchasing a genome sequencing exam that includes, testing, a follow-up physician consult, annual physician follow-up, and support services for various concerns and chronic diseases identified in the procedure. Research several providers to see who the best fit is; include Ancestry.com, Color Genomics, Helix, 23andMe, uBiome and any others you feel might work best for you. The Health-Wealth Personal Loss Assessment for Individuals will also prove beneficial in identifying other critical components individuals should prioritize.

UTILIZE ARTIFICIAL INTELLIGENCE, BLOCKCHAIN, AND MACHINE LEARNING TO IMPROVE YOUR HEALTH

SEVERAL YEARS AGO, I happened to be speaking at a healthcare event from the same stage as Dr. Tony Slonim, president and chief executive officer from Renown Health in Reno, Nevada. Renown Health includes multiple hospitals, physician groups, and health plans. Dr. Slonim made some ambitious predictions about the future of healthcare delivery during his speech. Having lived in northern Nevada for several years, I was intrigued and soaked it in.

Speaking together later in the day and having heard each other's talks, we found that we had much in common. Dr. Slonim said to me, "Dr. Luke, your vision is similar to mine and I am willing to try things in northern Nevada that aren't being done anywhere in America. We are just figuring out where to start!"

Dr. Slonim and I keep in touch and I have even offered up some support in some of his pioneering efforts at Renown. In 2017, I was pleased to learn of a new initiative Dr. Slonim had pioneered for Renown that focused on combining full genome sequencing and artificial intelligence. Met with initial enthusiasm, the initiative continued to expand with great success. Renown is creating enthusiasm and interest within in the local community for individuals to focus on the self-management of their personal health. Renown, as much an insurer as they are a hospital, is accomplishing what few other insurers have—getting individuals to take action to live healthier.

Within his first few years in the role, Dr. Slonim partnered with northern Nevada-based Desert Research Institute to find ways to use the institute's longstanding environmental data, and its impact on the citizens of Northern Nevada, to improve community health. One of their first steps was contacting the Nevada governor's office to request access to social data on Nevada citizens from the Governor's Office of Economic Development. They then partnered with DNA testing company 23andMe, and later partnered with Helix on the project.

The result of this project was a voluntary personalized medicine program designed to improve community health. The first day it was open to the public, the allotted 5,000 slots were all filled, so they immediately expanded the initiative to 10,000 voluntary slots which also filled to capacity quickly. The end result is a program that takes historical data, combines it with modern technology, and utilizes all new and real-time data to find out as much as possible about an individual in order to identify the best means to care for that person and maintain good health.

Artificial intelligence can be described in many ways, but as it pertains to human health and well-being it most often describes computer systems that have the ability to identify specific data points and coordinate with other computers or machines and perform various functions in a manner that traditionally required human interaction to complete. As a result, the computers and machines appear to possess intelligence. Think of artificial intelligence as machines searching, reading, learning, and comprehending data, and as a result making suggestions or providing analytical observations without any human interaction or involvement whatsoever. Northern Nevada's collaboration to improve community health has all the elements to gather data, to feed into computer systems that are designed to perform artificial intelligence, which as a result allows highly specialized personalized medicine.

The following are a few examples of how machine learning can be applied to developing healthcare analytics that have important repercussions for your own Health-Wealth future. Although the companies involved shared the following examples of work they are involved in, they asked me not to include their company names at this time, as these projects remain confidential as of this writing.

Our first example is from a company that has been experimenting with modifications to their employees' benefit offerings, attempting to motivate improved health behavior for covered employees and dependents. They offered to subsidize the acquisition of wearable technology to monitor activity level, basic physiological readings, and sleep habits. The offering of this option increased employee participation to nearly three times previous levels, but also required the employee to allow for analytics to be run on their de-identified data. After initiating these analytics, they found that they could coach their employees to sleep better by identifying personal behaviors, such as when to schedule exercise within their day. There may have been no direct correlation but there was a recognized improvement in overall health statistics for those employees who followed the guidance. This massive digital surveillance capability would not be financially feasible without the use of machine learning.

Another company, in this case a healthcare provider in an area affected by inversion layers that lead to environmentally exasperated breathing conditions, was challenged to effectively target which emergency units needed additional or reduced staffing based on the daily conditions. The search for information sources to guide decisions began with mining geo-tagged social media feeds for certain terms and phrases so they could identify prospective hot sites. Interestingly, as the basic model became refined, the health system started to get up to a four-hour head start on staffing requirements at their various facilities. Their findings demonstrate that the more data, machine learning, or artificial intelligence engines can ingest, the greater guidance and recommendations that can be provided.

This approach was further augmented with fully consented asthma registries, allowing for more understanding of where their most affected patients might be located. This moved the model from staffing to an early-warning method for those on the registry. The health system is now looking to do more of a crowd-sourcing model by issuing GPS-enabled inhalers and identify areas where the inhalers are being most used. This approach not only saves the health system money but improves health outcomes for all involved.

How might an individual benefit from AI, machine learning, and blockchain? Well, if you are paying attention, technology is everywhere. Remember how impressed you were the first time you typed in someone's email address and your computer recalled it on its own? That was only a few years ago—but now, you likely grow frustrated if your computer does not bring the email address up after you type the first few letters! That's an example of machine learning. Another example is when you jump in your car at a certain time of day and your car informs you that the traffic to your desired location is mild, even though you have not entered your destination. Your car seems to know where it's going based on the day of the week and time of day. These are examples of AI, machine learning, and blockchain at work.

How can your health benefit from similar advances? Paying attention to any and all data you encounter regarding your health is a great start. Remember it, record it, take a picture of it—put it to use for the health of it!

The possibilities are limitless, if you are willing to proactively contribute to the process. Numerous successful implementations have shown that data accumulation not only brings down the cost of care, it provides individuals with early warning and predictions about life-threatening diseases. Over time, technology will tell you what time of day is best for you to exercise, as well as the type of exercise and length of time you should exercise. For eating, nutrigenomics is rapidly developing so that individuals can learn which foods their body metabolizes more efficiently than others. It's no longer just as simple as calories, carbs, and fat grams; there is more to the weight loss game!

There are organizations offering consumer-centric, artificial intelligence programs. One industry leader, Betterpath, describes its platform as "harmonizing disparate healthcare activities simply by getting all of one's patient data in one place. It aligns past, present, and future data in an integrated record designed to provide patients, their caregivers, and their providers with information to manage and optimize care decisions." The data continues to accumulate over time to help identify personalized, outcomes-based interventions.

In 2019, Betterpath launched its first direct-to-consumer offering directly focused on connecting a person's wealth to his or her health. The Betterpath Savings Account connects personal finances and health data into an asset that consumers can use to both reduce the cost of their healthcare and earn meaningful income from their data. By rewarding people in cash for doing what's best for their health and allowing them to make money from their anonymized data, this "Savings Account" motivates consumers to take on the difficult task of health data collection and maintenance. Over time, Betterpath envisions using its AI platform to prove that this financial arbitrage structure (prospectively paying people to do what's best for their health) can actually save the health system significant costs in the long term.[15]

Great vehicles already exist for tracking the sort of data that companies like Betterpath are beginning to put to work. Many health plans offer a patient portal for you to track your own health. This is a great place to start tracking your health and lifestyle. These portals are largely built around information collected by the hospital and at a doctor's office. Over time, however, most portals are adding options for more lifestyle-based information as well.

Utilizing artificial intelligence, machine learning, and block-chain technology to improve your personal health is not as turnkey as other applications in this book, in that this requires you to pay attention and identify information as it becomes available. But if you follow through on the first two steps, and conduct physician consults to review your integrative medicine strategy and DNA test

---

15   From email correspondence with Betterpath CEO Matthew Sinderbrand, (September 11, 2018).

results, these are both great opportunities to seek out from the doctor what other data you should be keeping track of to improve health. Take the same approach at every doctor's appointment. When a doctor identifies a concern, ask where and how you might find and collect additional personal data on that topic as it emerges. Is it your smartphone, your wearable step monitor, Alexa, your car, or some other form of technology? Keep track of it all, and be conscious that everywhere you go, everywhere you look, your personal data is being collected. You can't challenge that collection, but you can put it to work Are you using your own data to your advantage?

UTILIZE TELEHEALTH AND REMOTE MONITORING SERVICES

I WAS SERVING AS THE EVENT EXECUTIVE CHAIR and emcee for the World Congress on Hospital Readmission Prevention in 2014 in Orlando, Florida. That same day, the event promoter was cohosting a separate event in the room next door, titled World Congress on Telehealth & Remote Monitoring. For the closing session, the two groups were combined, and I was asked along with the executive chair of the other event to deliver a closing keynote address to the combined crowd.

I presented first and was pleased with my delivery as I wrapped up and sat down. As I sat down in the crowd to hear the promoter's presentation, I thought it was odd that she was carrying a laptop onto the stage, walking slowly, and taking her time, as the technical team usually has the laptop ready to go. As she plugged in the laptop and logged on, she did not acknowledge the crowd. This dragged on for more than two minutes and became an almost uncomfortable silence. I grew nervous for my co-presenter.

Seconds later, onto her screen popped a video image of a man and a young boy. A few seconds later, the man said hello to the presenter in broken English, and she continued the conversation with him via her computer. She still had not addressed the crowd when she asked if she could examine the ear of the young boy next to him. The man on the screen grabbed the medical device used to examine the inner ear, gently placed it into the boy's ear, and there it was for the entire audience to see … a video image of the boy's inner ear, just as you would see in a doctor's office.

"Looks good," she said. "Now let me look at his throat please. How is he feeling?"

The man picked up another device and placed it in the boy's mouth. The entire audience then viewed the boy's throat. "He is feeling much better now, thank you," the man responded.

"Can you tell us the name of your clinic and where it's located," she said.

"Good Samaritan Clinic in Guatemala City, Guatemala," he replied.

A gasp was heard throughout the room. Her presentation was already impactful. What a simple, yet effective, approach to communicating the capabilities of modern-day medicine when telehealth and remote monitoring capabilities are applied. What we witnessed was not much more than the use of Skype and a few common medical-device cameras, yet we were all blown away. And this was in 2014! Why? We all used similar technology daily, but few organizations had applied it to care delivery at the time.

A lot has changed in the years since then. Technology has improved the speed and efficiency at which healthcare is delivered at a rapid pace in multiple ways. Nowhere is that more present than with the adoption of telehealth and remote monitoring capabilities.

Corporations throughout the country have realized that by providing a health plan that allows and encourages the use of telehealth appointments and remote monitoring capabilities can reduce time away from your family, treacherous minutes waiting in doctors waiting rooms, and waiting days for a doctor to fit you on the schedule. These mechanisms can reduce lost time at work and save you money as well!

A number of mobile applications are available that allow the patient and doctor to communicate through video on personal mobile phones or tablets. There are services that ensure a physician or NP is available at all times; appointments can be scheduled electronically, and "walk-in" time slots are often guaranteed for immediate access to a clinician who can remotely inspect the patient through video monitoring and then discuss the issues with the patient.

The rapid adoption of telehealth consults is one of the major drivers of the significantly reduced employer and employee spending reported by many companies that have converted to consumer-driven healthcare plans. Adoptions that save your employer money can save you money, too!

Once your corporate health plan allows and promotes remote physician consults, try it out as soon as you are able. Although many individuals are initially skeptical, once you have consulted a doctor from your phone, tablet, or computer, you may not ever want to go sit and wait in a doctor's office again! This is the exact manner in which residents of island communities or rural areas—or our patient in Guatemala—have been conducting virtual consults for years. Heck, I even tried it myself—and I am sold!

In the summer of 2018, I went to the doctor twice, as my head was congested. The doctor (well, truth be told the nurse practitioner serving at a drug store's urgent care facility) kept telling me it was a cold and I did need not medication. I then went out of town and became convinced I had a sinus infection. While traveling, I signed up on the app through my phone with Lemonaid Health. com. Within fifteen minutes I had enrolled in their program, and just a few minutes after my enrollment was complete a doctor (a real MD this time) popped onto my computer screen and consulted me. Within ten minutes the doctor prescribed medicine to me for a sinus infection and had the prescription filled to my pharmacy of choice. (Next-day delivery to my home was also offered as an option). I was impressed.

When researching Lemonaid Health, you will see that they offer twenty-five-dollar online doctor consultations and promote rapid delivery of medication. Medications they are able to prescribe regularly treat conditions including acid reflux, acne, birth control, cholesterol tests, erectile dysfunction, hair loss, lab tests, sinus infection, smoking cessation, and urinary tract infection. In many cases, the entire registration, consult, medication cost, and processing fee is less than sixty dollars. This is just one example of a non-traditional approach to utilizing technology via telemedicine and finding alternative sources for medication-fulfillment at affordable prices.

Similarly, remote monitoring devices are being deployed routinely for a number of common chronic diseases, as well as other health needs. Seniors battling congestive heart failure are often provided a Bluetooth scale, as sudden weight loss or gain can be an early indication of complications, so when they weigh in every day, the result is electrically reported. If there is a significant loss or gain, the patient's insurer, physician, or clinical case manager is automatically notified. Other examples of remote monitors are devices that monitor heart rate or devices that send an alert each time a patient stands up or sits down. The capabilities of remote devices in improving care are endless.

As employers address chronic disease through value bundles and other coordinated programs, remote monitoring devices are almost always one of the tactics included in the care plan. The cost of many of these devices has come down significantly. At least seven of the eleven steps to Health-Wealth in some manner include a component of telehealth or remote monitoring. This illustrates how beneficial this approach can be in reducing wasteful spending.

There are a number of providers available to consumers and businesses that simplify this process. One example is ReadyDoc MD, which is a bundle of valuable services, one service provider being market leader Teladoc. Teladoc is a nationwide network of highly qualified doctors who can diagnose, recommend treatment, and prescribe medication when necessary through phone or video consultations. ReadyDoc MD (www.doconthego.net) utilizes the Teladoc network to bring to life the vast resources offered to simplify getting access to a physician and do so at a much lower price and in a more timely and convenient manner. This partnership, for example, can reduce unnecessary visits to the doctor by offering quality health-care consultations in minutes by phone, video, or mobile app, often with no co-pays or deductibles, depending on an employer's benefit plan. ReadyDoc MD is available direct to the consumer by visiting the website.

In summary, individuals should consider a health plan that allows and promotes remote and virtual visits, provides mobile applications and hopefully, offers no co-pay or reduced co-pay for you if you choose to conduct a virtual visit as opposed to one in person. Save money. Save time. Utilizing telehealth does not require much convincing for millennials and Gen Z, as they grew up with the technology in their hands. Gen Xers and baby boomers though, sometimes need a little push to try something new, especially when it is technology based and personal.

No matter your age, let this book be the nudge you need to give a remote physician consult a try!

PARTICIPATE IN LOCAL MEDICAL TOURISM

DO YOU REMEMBER IN CHAPTER 2 when we identified all of the villains of greed in the healthcare delivery system? Hospitals, insurers, Big Pharma, etc.? Now is the time for you to apply pressure to the villains of greed, specifically your local hospital!

Before I became a hospital executive, my wife and I were trying to decide which hospital we would choose to deliver our third child. Our insurance opted for either of our two top choices. Both were local, one a big, shiny medical center and one small boutique community hospital. My wife immediately suggested the big, shiny hospital. I had just started a new job and preferred a small hospital where I could pop in and out of the parking lot for a few days with relative ease, and more importantly, my wife and child would be among the only individuals in the small unit during their stay. Just as it should be: my two top girls would be treated like royalty by the nurses!

Our insurance carrier advised that we were free to deliver at either. But to prepare financially, I called each hospital in advance to confirm what our share of costs would be. After all, this is capitalism, right? "Maybe I can play the hospitals against each other and get a discount like I do car dealers," I thought. No such luck.

When I called to inquire about prices, I got the same answer from both. Prices? You are kidding, right?! Why would we have a price sheet? Just because every other business in the country shares their prices in advance, why would you think a hospital would do that?!? In fact, many industries, including those in the financial and real estate sectors, are required by law to secure signed, written confirmation of prices in advance. But hospitals, no way!

So, I drove to the community hospital around the corner from my house and personally requested a price sheet. I once again was told that the hospital did not have a pricing sheet, and that even if they did, it would be an estimate, as it all depends on what the doctor and hospital staff chose to code and bill for during the procedure.

At that point, I asked to speak with the hospital business office manager. This is before I had ever worked a day in any hospital, so this was all new to me. When the manager emerged, she used the eight words that I now refer to as the "Eight Words that Killed American Healthcare." She said, not to concern myself with pricing, "Don't worry, your insurance will pay for it."

Little did I know at the time she was giving me false hope and made me feel that because my share of costs at the time of delivery were fixed, that any additional costs to my company would almost certainly be passed back onto me in the following yearly renewal. Here's a word of advice based on this experience: when you are an employee covered by employer-sponsored insurance, choose the higher-cost hospital, even though the price might not be greater for you at the time, it will directly impact the amount of money you and your fellow employees have to pay the following year. If your health insurance is provided by your company, ask the benefits manager or human resources department to discuss options and prices in advance of a procedure so you are educated on the prices and total costs. Although hospitals are often hesitant to share prices with consumers, health plans contractually require hospitals to share procedure prices with contracted employers, so employers can keep them on file. In essence, it's "fool's gold" to believe that your insurance will pay for it. A more appropriate description would be "deferred payment." Deferred until next year!

We covered the lack of hospital transparency earlier in the book, so you get the point. But now it's time for you to act. Want to save $5,000 in one year on healthcare? This may be your chance; choose the right hospital! It's called Local Medical Tourism. Shop!

Guess what? Your company may offer a deep discount for services performed at a center of excellence in Costa Rica, India, or Las Vegas. But it also likely has options just a few miles away from your home as well! Why is Local Medical Tourism important? Because the cost can fluctuate significantly from local providers who are not centers of excellence. In fact, the complete cost of all-inclusive care could be less than $15,000, instead of $80,000 at your local provider.

How is this possible? As we have discussed, there is no accountability or justification in hospital pricing in the United States because each hospital sets its own rates, and the variance is significant. There is no reason to believe any accountability is on the horizon, either. Hospitals, surgery centers, and independent practices have the ability to set their own rates and charge significantly less than many larger hospitals, which is why medical tourism can exist even from one county to the next. If you don't shop, you will never know.

Thus, the opening of many new medical tourism-focused companies abroad is just one sign that medical tourism has seen explosive growth since 2008. Medical tourism continues to grow in popularity, as the average cost of care can be drastically lessened by simply getting on an airplane and traveling to a destination. Consider this: the employer pays for airfare and four nights' accommodations for an employee and one guest, then covers the cost of care. Using the example cited earlier, with a $5,000 travel budget for the employee and guest plus a $15,000 all-inclusive procedure, the employer's total spend is $20,000, in comparison to $60,000 or $80,000 had the employee received the care locally, even if they had chosen a local center of value. Even after travel expenses, the company often saves more than 50 percent of the potential cost.

Medical tourism can even refer to the town next door, not just the other side of the globe. If you think about it, this concept of going out of market, whether just a few miles or thousands of miles, is completely backwards. The local providers have the complete ability to lower costs and compete, they just don't have any financial incentive to do so, so they continue to raise prices aggressively.

Because Americans have been slower to acclimate to international medical tourism than employers had hoped, many employers have simply looked to the next town to find a hospital that will partner with them to be a center of value. Referring back to the individual employee savings in the example earlier in the chapter, would you be willing to drive an extra thirty-five miles for a procedure for you or a family member if it saved you $1,800 or more?

In 2017, Santa Barbara County in California announced it was going to take all of its hip surgeries to San Diego County, a three-hour drive to the south. This decision was not driven by a shortage of doctors or hospitals in Santa Barbara; in fact, Cottage Health in

Santa Barbara has multiple hospitals and a great reputation. Apparently, the county was able to negotiate a significant discount by shopping the contract out of the county. Once they showed that the quality scores were just as strong at the other hospital, as well as how much less patients would pay in their share of cost, the program was an easy sell.

Most Americans have read about or heard about medical tourism. But few have ever been willing to fly to another country to receive healthcare services, even if the cost was significantly less, sometimes even 75 percent or so cheaper. The discounted price was not enough to invoke behavioral change in the majority of Americans. While international medical tourism is still an extremely viable option in regard to saving significant healthcare dollars, local medical tourism within the United States has proven to be a much more popular option than seeking services internationally.

In fact, most medical tourism is within the same state where you reside. Social media influencer and longtime health insurance broker David Contorno jumped the state line for his procedure. Although Contorno flew from North Carolina to Oklahoma for a procedure that he documented in a social media video, he estimates that most people who choose to participate in local medical tourism are driving less than thirty-five miles to find the center of excellence that offers them the same or better quality, at a much more attractive price. Thirty-five miles!

"When I show an employer how there is frequently much better care at a significantly lower price that may be outside their familiar local market, they often feel their employees would never travel for health care," said David Contorno, founder of E Powered Benefits, when I interviewed him. "I ask them if they thought their employees would drive four hours to pick up a new car from a dealership that was $100 less per month on the payment, and they all say yes, with a pretty quick awareness how much more willing we should be to go to wherever the best place of care is going to be, at the lowest cost."

Great example!

The best thing you as a consumer can do to combat unjustifiably inflated hospital and physician costs is to shop in advance. Just like you would shop for a car or a house, compare prices. Remember the story in chapter 6 about taking your hypothetical daughter shopping for a car? Well, we have arrived at the moment of truth. Which way are you going to turn?

Seek out "in-network" providers, but do not stop there. Seek out true centers of excellence, compare prices, compare quality, and do your homework. Ask friends, post questions on social media seeking recommendations and reviews, and approach your employer to confirm you are utilizing all of the resources at your disposal. Your employer should be making a list of centers of excellence readily available to you.

With the growing popularity of high deductible plans among employers, it's likely you are paying for a significant chunk of any hospital procedure or stay, so shopping in advance is definitely in your best interest.

Employers are more frequently referring employees to centers of excellence, specifically for high-cost procedures including hip replacement, back surgery, fertility, and bariatrics. In 2013, Walmart and several other major employers went so far as to contract with only four hospitals nationwide to serve as centers of excellence to perform free (to the employee) hip and knee replacements. Employees could still choose local providers, but then they would have to pay for the procedure themselves.[16] In fact, in 2017, almost 50 percent of Walmart employees' hip replacement surgeries were performed at centers of excellence, up from approximately 40 percent in 2016. The point here is simple: price matters, and quality care is available at centers of excellence.

Use all the resources at your disposal to make an educated and financially responsible decision driven by pricing information, quality data, patient-satisfaction data, word of mouth, and proximity. More often than not there is a center of excellence available to you within your own community, at a significantly less expensive cost than simply going with the biggest hospital in town because you perceive it to be better. Do the research; you are likely to find that the quality at the alternative facility, the center of excellence, is the same or better.

Demand price transparency from the hospital, as they DO have the prices to provide you when you ask and demand them, and new rules implemented in 2018 require hospitals to more proactively post prices—so shop and compare prices offered by other hospitals, local surgery centers, imaging centers or labs. Share pricing with the hospital you prefer and see if they will match competitor's prices. Ask for the cash rate for a procedure in addition to how much your share of cost through insurance will be. Other options include requesting a payment plan, cash discount, or pay-in-full upfront discount.

Remember, a good test to see if the hospital is transparent to begin with is by asking them to share their procedure prices in advance. And this should improve, as in 2018 federal legislation passed implementing financial penalties for hospitals that do not post prices.

---

16   "NBGH/Optimum: Culture of Health Study," National Business Group on Health, accessed November 28, 2017.

But don't forget the ol' company line I was taught as a hospital administrator, "It's just an estimate: our doctors and nurses decide what to bill for during the procedure." The kicker is you are likely under anesthesia when they are performing the procedure, so you have no means to determine what procedures and supplies were actually used! And you are completely helpless and have no means of recourse to debate what the hospital bills for!

Go online and seek out others who have sought a more affordable approach to the same procedure you are faced with. Seek out resources like the federal government's "CMS Compare" website (www.cms.gov) that compares hospital and physician quality scores. While it's not perfect, it's the chosen methodology and a valuable resource. Use it! There are private companies like TopCare, managed by my respected friend Jeff Bernhard, that also provide a hospital and physician comparison platform available to payers, companies, and individuals. Ask your employer if they have any resources to compare the quality of doctors and hospitals.

Once you shop and choose a center of excellence, don't stop there. Hold the hospital accountable. Review the bill line by line. Ask for confirmation and evidence that the invoice is accurate. You would be amazed at how often hospitals bills include errors and overcharges. I am comfortable saying it is "more often than not" that a hospital bill includes an error. Call them on it, ask for a refund when confirmed!

Let me challenge and inspire you to take on your local hospital when you are caught up in the system that is broken beyond repair! When you get an outrageous invoice for share of costs from the hospital, call and negotiate with them. Find out if what your insurance has already paid exceeds their cash rate. Then ask them to waive the balance and your share of costs. It's worth a try. Copy your local congressman on all correspondence. Also, research who sits on the hospital's community board of directors and copy them on correspondence or take them for coffee to discuss your concerns as well.

Many hospitals won't negotiate with you until you are sent to a collection agency. Let me expose a well-kept secret. In many cases, hospitals actually own the collection agency. They just brand it under a different name and locate it off campus so there are separate addresses. Other hospitals simply sell the debt to a collection agency for ten cents on the dollar and have no further incentive to assist them in collecting it from you. Also, are you aware that medical bills are not reportable on your credit report? All things to keep in mind when it's time to negotiate. You need all the bargaining power you can get!

Whenever a medical organization threatens to send me to collections, I always ask them if they can please do so right away "so I can negotiate with them, since you won't negotiate with me!" That always throws them off. But wait, the phone operator is the very person who told me they were not allowed to negotiate, that prices were firm based on what was billed. Well, that is true until it's passed to collections. Request they send it directly to collections! Hey, it's worked for me several times, and it's fun to hear how they react. You're taking away the phone operator's ability to threaten you with collections, and they weren't trained to handle that!

And for goodness sake, when the hospital sends you a fluffy, feel-good mailer asking for charitable donations for their new building project or holiday fundraiser, just remember who the number one villain of greed is (in chapter 2 of this book), and that you may still have an outstanding bill for that same hospital for a basic procedure that likely cost them less than 20 percent of what they are charging you.

Do yourself a favor; start shopping for healthcare just like you do for shoes.

ENROLL IN DISEASE-SPECIFIC VALUE PROGRAMS

DID YOU KNOW THAT approximately 5 percent of individuals account for more than 50 percent of overall healthcare spending?[17] What if you or one of your family members number among that 5 percent of high utilizers? Well, that could be why you bought this book!

There are now a number of companies nationwide that provide programs to significantly reduce spending on chronic conditions or high-cost services for individuals in need, who ultimately account for the majority of overall healthcare spending.

---

17   Karen Weintraub and Rachel Zimmerman, "Fixing the 5 Percent," *The Atlantic, June 29, 2017, https://www.theatlantic.com/health/archive/2017/06/fixing-the-5-percent/532077/.*

A recent study noted that 60 percent of American adults have at least one chronic condition, and more than 40 percent have more than one chronic condition.[18]

Respected, longtime healthcare executive and recently retired Dartmouth-Hitchcock CEO Dr. James Weinstein shared in 2017 that he had identified nine critical ideas for changing healthcare. One of those nine ideas was to focus on the top 5 percent of healthcare users.[19] That is the focus of this rule.

Common high-cost diseases, procedures, and surgeries include hip and knee replacement, back surgery, fertility treatment, cancer treatment, and cardiac care. Several complications commonly associated with obesity, including diabetes and bariatric surgery, are also common high-cost services. Are you or a family member impacted by any of these?

In recent years, several companies have emerged that are providing specialized programs to individuals impacted by these diseases and symptoms that provide significant savings to the individual and family. The models differ slightly, but all have the same goal of reducing healthcare spending while enhancing access and care for a handful of specific, high-cost procedures and complications.

One approach to identifying savings is often referred to as *specialized wraparound coverage.* Organizations like Hixme offer a variety of plans and actually allow different family members to enroll in various disease-specific plans. Hixme claims to have "right-fitting" coverage for each individual and also offers partner hospital options

---

18   Ayla Ellison, "41% of healthcare spending attributed to 12% of Americans, study finds," *Becker's Hospital Review, May 30, 2017, https://www.beckershospitalreview.com/finance/41-of-healthcare-spending-attributed-to-12-of-americans-study-finds.html.*

19   Molly Gamble, "Dartmouth-Hitchcock CEO Dr. James Weinstein: 'If we had to redesign healthcare today, it wouldn't look anything like it does now' — 9 ideas for change," *Becker's Hospital Review, May 23, 2017, https://www.beckershospitalreview.com/hospital-management-administration/dartmouth-hitchcock-ceo-dr-james-weinstein-if-we-had-to-redesign-healthcare-today-it-wouldn-t-look-anything-like-it-does-now-9-ideas-for-change.html.*

and similar ways for individuals to utilize centers of excellence for additional savings.

Canary Health offers programs in diabetes management, stress management, and caregiver training. It also offers a self-management program that assists with arthritis, heart disease, and depression. Canary Health, which created a Diabetes Prevention Program and a Chronic Disease Self-Management Program, claims it has reduced diabetes cases by approximately 80 percent, with residual additional savings as a result of reduced emergency department and physician office utilization.

Livongo is another company that partners with individuals to better manage diabetes. Livongo's digital platform is combined with coaching to effectively manage diabetes and keep unnecessary spending down. Omada Health also offers a digital platform that serves as a self-management platform for weight loss, which subsequently reduces risk for type 2 diabetes, stroke, and heart disease. Omada claims its participants lower their diabetes risk by 30 percent and their likelihood for stroke by more than 15 percent.

Though much attention is placed on wellness programs and management of chronic diseases like diabetes and heart disease, individuals should not neglect the impact of musculoskeletal disorders. For example, PeerWell, a technology company based in San Francisco, has developed a comprehensive program, PreHab, to aid patients awaiting orthopedic surgery. PreHab is an evidence-based program designed to optimize a person's health profile to the specific surgery he or she will have. The program offers methods to improve a range of health factors, including exercise, nutrition, social and environment preparation, and anxiety and pain management leading up to surgery. The proprietary PreHab program allows patients to go home faster and perform rehabilitation and recovery from the comfort of their homes, leading to an estimated $2,900 per person in additional savings.

PeerWell's program has become a must-have among patients. Patients from all over the country are proactively seeking out PreHab to improve their surgery experiences and take on more self-care. Employers can do more than they are doing to improve the healthcare experience for their employees struggling with musculoskeletal disorders and can offer solutions to get them back on their feet, feeling pain-free, and able to engage meaningfully in their work.

"Musculoskeletal disorders effect 50 percent of adults and are the leading cause of claims costs by employer-sponsored health plans in the US today," said Manish Shah, CEO of PeerWell in emails we exchanged. "Much of this cost is driven by surgery, imaging, and prescription medications. In addition, employers need to account for lower productivity, absenteeism, and increased disability and workers compensation insurance premiums. Programs like PeerWell and others can bend the cost curve, improve outcomes, and improve satisfaction."

What if you are not a high utilizer of healthcare resources but are still willing to put in the additional time and effort to improve your health and lifestyle? There are programs for you as well. They are often paid for by the employer. For example, Marquee Health offers the employer-sponsored Marquee Health Nurse Health Coaching Program for its employees. The program is designed to work with employees to establish goals based on individual health needs, and a nurse is provided to provide support and assist employees in achieving those goals.[20]

Marquee Health has a Nurse Coach, for example, who works in partnership with the patient's physician. Common areas of focus are

---

20   For more information, visit www.marqueehealth.com.

guidance and recommendations on diet, stress reduction, physical activity, medication review and management, and reduction of tobacco use. The program is often available to all employees, but specializes in catering to the same high-cost chronic conditions discussed throughout this section, including: asthma, chronic kidney disease, chronic pain, congestive heart failure, coronary artery disease, diabetes, high cholesterol, and high blood pressure among others. Similar supplemental programs are available throughout the country. For example, Catapult Health promotes itself as preventative care and claims it requires "no deductibles and no co-pays." An attractive offering for those looking for guidance on improving lifestyle but who do not necessarily have the budget to pay for such guidance.

There are more programs too numerous to mention here, but there is one common thread in each: the patient must engage in order to benefit from these programs. These programs are diverse, have wide-ranging price points, and are not always a great fit for everyone based on individual needs. However, knowing which company is the best fit for you or your family member is a critical and complicated first step, as each provider is unique. The Health-Wealth Personal Loss Assessment was designed to identify which program is the most appropriate fit for you or your family.

Once you complete the Health-Wealth Personal Loss Assessment, research each option to see which is the best fit and if they offer direct to consumer programs. If the provider does not offer direct-to-consumer programs, request the contact information so you can take it to your human resources department to sign up! The good news is that if you take this approach, even though it may take a little longer to set up, your company will likely get a discount and may even pay for the entire program for you.

When it comes to controlling healthcare costs, one of the most effective tactics is quantifying your most expensive needs, identifying common chronic issues and high-cost procedures, and developing specialty programs to more effectively manage that family member's health. This discussion has shared just a handful of programs available to support you in this process.

Although these bundling approaches may seem laborious and complicated to facilitate, they can actually be one of the simplest and quickest tactics to implement that lead to significant savings. The resources and organizations that manage these programs on your behalf specialize in these services and were created to better care for individuals with chronic diseases.

CONVERT TO A PLAN OFFERING DIRECT PRIMARY CARE

INDIVIDUALS WHO HAVE CONVERTED to direct primary care (DPC) plans are reporting much greater satisfaction with DPC than in their traditional PPO or HMO. The primary reason is that doctors are spending two-to-three times longer with patients during office visits than in prior models. It's the return of the primary care physician, the reinvention of the patient/doctor relationship in many cases!

DPC is one of the most rapidly emerging models being employed and is likely to continue gaining momentum for several years to come, as it is proving to save money for businesses providing commercial insurance and also improving patient access and satisfaction.

DPC is a value-based primary care model that increases operational efficiency and doctor-patient satisfaction while reducing overhead by cutting out the middleman, insurance, and a lot of the red tape and bureaucracy from healthcare. In short, DPC medical practices do not accept any form of insurance. Employers and employees are enrolled in an exchange that pays the physician a per-patient monthly retainer fee. This retainer fee most often ranges from $50–$100 a month per patient (the employer pays a portion and you pay the rest). In exchange, the individual is entitled to a specified set of services offered by the physician or practice.

How does DPC differ from a concierge practice? Concierge products are more often premium services that are significantly more expensive than $100 a month. Concierge medical practices often accept insurance but also charge a yearly membership for immediate access. Concierge practices are more like VIP or country club medicine, prominent in affluent communities where access to physicians is sparse or long wait times to see a doctor are an issue. This is not the case with the DPC model.

Aside from the financial benefits listed below, DPC has already enhanced access to the diminishing availability of primary care in many affected markets. Further, DPC is restoring the accountability of doctors when it comes to fulfilling the needs of their patients, and it reduces the administrative burden of many traditional insurance policies. DPC doctors claim they spend much more time with patients, often advertising up to thirty minutes of direct physician access per appointment. Because each DPC practice's entire book of patients is often smaller than those of practices accepting insurance, doctors have more time for patient interaction and involvement in individual care planning. This additional time spent on care planning allows the physician to better communicate and explain why traditionally routine follow-up tests, exams, and referrals are not needed.

With the extra time spent with patients, together they can discover ways to live a healthy lifestyle and optimize well-being.

Kat Quinn, a patient advocate for MyDPC.org, shared in a personal interview, "One of the best perks about DPC is that many DPC practices offer wellness programs that are included in the membership fee, like yoga, tai chi, nutrition workshops, and more to promote a healthy lifestyle."

Benefits of the DPC model include a stronger patient/doctor relationship, the reestablishing of the personal family physician, and enhanced access to the services offered by the doctor or medical practice. Since you are paying a retainer fee, the doctor has stronger incentives to shorten wait times, improve customer service, and keep patients satisfied. That kind of sounds like the way things used to be, doesn't it?

As a matter of fact, Generation Xers were the first to experience the dissipation of the patient-doctor relationship, as the days of the personal family physician started going by the wayside in the 1970s and 1980s. The 1980s brought an expansion of HMOs, and health insurance largely became reactionary and focused more on catastrophic events. Year over year, the routine, annual health physical became less and less of a priority to American citizens.

There are other ways that DPC can save you money as well. DPC doctors minimize ordering unnecessary tests, exams, and specialty referrals and will often only refer patients to specialists who are preferred providers or centers of excellence that offer a discounted rate for the initial consult. The model actually puts the primary care doctors to work for you, incentivizing them to assist you in reducing avoidable spending on unnecessary services, which were so often ordered and abused in the FFS model. This additional physician time and access is a critical component of operating a successful DPC model. Each model inevitably differs slightly to best meet the specific needs of each community, but enhanced access to physicians, shorter wait times, and longer face time with the physician are the common thread.

"We are working to create win-win onsite clinics and DPC models for as many small and mid-size businesses as we are large corporations," said Mike Ochoa, Founder of Transcend Onsite Care which has successful collaborations in both California and Texas, when we spoke together. "Transcend is also unique in that we combine a pharmacy benefit manager, Ascend PBM, into the DPC model for our clients for additional savings as well."

Employers who have converted to a DPC model—for the most part—have seen overall spending come down twenty to 30 percent on average.[21] Those savings are being passed on to the employee.

This overall savings is a result of DPC practices being incentivized to keep overall spending down and focusing on the following items:

- Reducing unnecessary specialist referrals.

- Avoiding ordering unnecessary exams, labs, and medications.

- Referring only to specialists and ancillary providers who guarantee a discounted rate for the employer and employee.

- Avoiding unnecessary referrals to the emergency department.

- Avoiding unnecessary hospital referrals.

- Prescribing generic, affordable medications as often as possible.

---

21   For more information, visit www.marqueehealth.com.

With all this considered, it is important to understand that your employer will essentially be offering two separate insurance policies to each employee: a primary care policy (DPC) and a catastrophic policy (for all else).

Remember, in the FFS model doctors were financially incentivized in multiple ways to order exams, tests, hospitalizations, and expensive medications, even when unnecessary. It was almost a "don't ask, don't tell" approach, meaning that the less the doctor finds out about your situation, the more justification he or she has to over-utilize and order unnecessary exams that generate additional revenue for the practice. DPC removes these incentives, which are in direct contrast to the employer's desire to reduce spending on healthcare.

Many of the services in the DPC policy are offered at no cost. For example, the savings on routine tests and wellness checks alone ranges from $35-$450 per procedure for the services listed below.

- Twenty-four-hour access to physician or NP

- Allergy injections

- Annual exam

- Annual Pap test

- Chronic care management

- Blood draws

- EKGs

- Flu shots

- Lab tests

- Management of hospital and specialist referrals

- Nebulizer treatments

- Pregnancy tests

- School and youth sports physicals

- Spirometry

- Strep tests

- Urine tests

- Urgent care

- X-rays (imaging)

DPC cuts down your costs by offering each of these services at no cost to members. Further, although not free, the savings offered on routine lab work and prescriptions can be significant, as illustrated by the chart below.

MEMBER LAB TEST SAVINGS

Test	Member Price	Average Retail Price
CBC	$4.00	$50.00
CMP	$5.00	$50.00
Lipids	$5.00	$90.00
PSA	$10.00	$60.00
TSH	$7.00	$95.00
HgbA1C	$5.00	$50.00

Source: Blue Skies Family Medicine

MEMBER PRESCRIPTION SAVINGS

Medication	Member Price	Retail Pharmacy/ GoodRx Cost
Amoxicillin	$1.70	$10.00
Celexa	$1.11	$4.00
Flonase	$8.10	$15.20
Imitrex	$11.59	$20.25
Lipitor	$4.14	$19.00
Metformin	$1.11	$4.00
Singulair	$5.04	$35.00
Z-Pak	$7.82	$15.00

Source: Blue Skies Family Medicine

There are several major insurance carriers that offer paired packages of DPC coverage along with a high-deductible plan for emergencies, niche services, and catastrophic coverage.

Allow me to financially quantify this opportunity. At present, most companies spend about five percent of their total healthcare spending on primary care. By converting to a DPC model, a company is more likely to spend in excess of 10 percent on primary care, as they are converting to a subscription model of sorts. With that said, at the end of the month and year, the company's overall healthcare spending will likely drop by at least 20 percent due to reduced utilization. Typically, when your employee wins, you win when it comes to healthcare savings.

The ultimate goal in reading this book is to identify tactics that could be implemented to save your family on its overall healthcare spend. Converting to DPC accomplishes this by spending a higher percentage of your dollars on primary care. In my experience, primary care physicians' decisions can affect up to 90 percent of your overall healthcare spending. So why not align incentives? As a result of this enhanced pipeline to a physician, your family is often healthier and happier.

Although this book focuses almost entirely on individual turnkey tactics to reduce spending for you or your family, DPC is one tactic that is an exception to this turnkey approach. Finding a DPC provider may require you to either shop plans or lean on your employer as the provider of insurance to implement this model. If your company has 400 or more employees in your location, or 500 or more in the local area, then this model could be ideal for your company to implement. If you do not have the option of a DPC, I encourage you talk with your employer and help educate them on savings they could realize.

USE ALTERNATIVE APPROACHES TO BUYING MEDICATION

THERE HAS TO BE A MORE AFFORDABLE WAY to buy medications, right? Well, sometimes, but remember, the Big Pharma lobbying budget is the largest of any industry in the country.

Consider this story from Bloomberg in 2018. Iowa pharmacist Mark Frahm noticed something unusual as he compared a newspaper notice with his own records. Frahm saw that for a bottle of generic antipsychotic pills, CVS had billed Wapello County $198.22. But his company, South Side Drug was reimbursed just $5.73.

"So why was CVS charging almost $200 for a bottle of pills that it told the pharmacy was worth less than six dollars? And what was the company doing with the other $192.49? Frahm had stumbled across what's known as spread pricing, where companies like CVS markup—sometimes dramatically—the difference between the amount they reimburse pharmacies for a drug and the amount they charge their clients. It's where pharmacy benefit managers (PBMs) like CVS make a part of their profit. But Frahm says he didn't think the spread could be thousands of percent."[22]

So, now that you have heard that story, how would you approach the issue if you were an employee of Wapello County? Would you tell your employer that you would order the drugs on your own from your local pharmacy? Would you let your employer know that by doing so you are saving yourself significant dollars, as well as the company? Would you ask your employer to pay your share of costs to the pharmacy even though the pharmacy might charge a twenty-five dollar co-pay instead of the normal ten dollars? Would you ask your employer to pick up the additional fifteen-dollar difference if you could show them that even they could likely save $120 on the prescription as a result of spread pricing?

Why wouldn't you? And your company would be smart to consider it!

Recent reports show that Healthcare Lobbying Expenses exceed $713 Million annually,[23] which includes Big Pharma, insurance carriers, hospitals, HMOs and providers combined. Of that $713 million, $279 annually is from Big Pharma lobbying alone, which makes it the largest lobby in DC.

Then there is Walmart. Walmart offers generic drugs for one dollar and five dollars. Here's a quick tip for you. Anytime you are prescribed a medicine by a doctor, immediately ask them if there is a generic option or an alternative should your insurance not cover the

---

22 Robert Langreth, David Ingold, and Jackie Gu, "The Secret Drug Pricing System Middlemen Use to Rake in Millions", *Bloomberg*, accessed September 11, 2018.

23 Michael Chandler, Seeking Alpha, accessed June 14, 2018, https://seekingalpha.com/author/michael-chandler#regular_articles.

prescribed medication or if the co-pay is too high. This should become part of your routine anytime a doctor prescribes you medication.

Some companies offer mail order medication options that can reduce your share of costs as well. Most companies nationwide have partnered with programs to assist them in reducing costs for medications. Thus, it would be wise for anyone covered by employer provided insurance to acquire with the benefits manager or human resources manager to ensure you are aware of the most cost-efficient approach to ordering medication. These programs are particularly impactful.

For someone with a chronic disease that has a long-term projection of medication consumption, especially when it is a premium product and the medication and co-pay are expensive. In fact, if you or a family member is subject to an ongoing long-term medication for a chronic disease, this rule is likely your quickest route to health-wealth savings. I may not list the program that is your direct answer in this chapter, but the point is that, if a good portion of your budget is going to pay for medication at present, speak to your corporate benefits manager, work your friends on social media, research less expensive options for securing the medication and start saving money. I promise, there is a solution out there.

Corporations are becoming wise to the under-the-table tactics of Big Pharma, and they are acting. Many corporations are contracting with providers like Euphora Health and California-based Carrum Health, who connect employers directly to top-performing providers to assist in medication management.[24] Such approaches essentially replace the PBM with a new middleman whose entire role is to find

---

24   PwC Health Research Institute, "Top health industry issues of 2018: A year for resilience and uncertainty," 2018, https://www.pwc.com/us/en/industries/health-industries/top-health-industry-issues.html.

you the most cost-effective medication. So, we are moving in the right direction.

As this brief discussion can help you see, there are many steps that can be taken to rein in pharmacy spending. These are four examples of tactics that can significantly your spending on medications:

1. Choose a plan that offers generic drugs completely free.

2. Ask for generics or alternatives to high-priced drugs.

3. Seek access to discount plans including mail-in, Walmart, or others.

4. Utilize technology such as telehealth to get access to doctors and suppliers who are able to prescribe and supply more affordable drugs.

While my experience was with Lemonaid Health (described in step number five), there are plenty of other options available to you throughout the country. Do some research in your region and with your employer; ask your doctor and nurse to identify which are programs are available to you, which are most popular, and if there are any specific to your area. Before you research, invest the time and money in completing Health-Wealth step number two: getting your DNA test done. You must learn how your body metabolizes different medications before you can effectively utilize medications that are both effective and cost efficient.

HEALTH-WEALTH FOR WOMEN

THERE ARE A NUMBER OF PROGRAMS and applications emerging in recent years that have had a significant impact on the Health-Wealth of women. Led by the Maven clinic, below is a partial list of several applications that are popular with women in improving health, reducing lost time from work, and reducing overall wasteful healthcare spending.

Katherine Ryder founded Maven Clinic in New York to make health practitioners across the country more accessible to women. Maven provides a platform for on-demand physician appointments for women and targets active, busy women. Maven is a digital clinic where women communicate via telehealth with healthcare providers including doctors, nutritionists, gynecologists, midwives, and psychologists, among other practitioners. Maven has a mobile app that also features a forum that allows the community to connect and share experiences.

Spruce is a telehealth platform focused specifically on skin. Although Spruce is not specific to females, it's much more popular with women than men. Similar to my Lemonaid Health experience, you are asked to first complete a brief personal questionnaire. Then you are consulted by a dermatologist and a treatment plan. Spruce charges a forty-dollar fee, and in addition to the initial appointment it includes thirty days of follow-up questions and a follow-up appointment. Spruce will also submit prescriptions on your behalf. With a national shortage of dermatologists making it difficult to get an appointment, Spruce has seen rapid growth.

Clementine is a hypnotherapy application designed to help women feel confident. Clementine focuses on four key areas to relieve stress in women—sleep, confidence, de-stress, and mantras—and has proven beneficial for those who have utilized it. Clementine features a confidence-boost session and challenges you to describe what success looks like to you in your own words. Starting with visualization and a focus on imagery, the guide then progresses to goal-setting and forming an action plan. A constant theme is to shake off issues that arise and stay focused on your goals. You are able to select a session based on how you are feeling, and there is another feature that is simply a recording for five minutes when an individual may need to "take a breather."

Glow is one of several programs designed to best manage a woman's menstrual cycle and includes an ovulation calculator that records a woman's period, mood, symptoms, sex, and medication. Glow is free and includes cycle charts and weight monitoring and birth control reminders. Like Maven, Glow includes a popular chat feature so users can compare notes. Glow also syncs with other health devices and apps including Fitbit, Jawbone, and MyFitnessPal.

Clue is another app designed specifically to improve women's health through their menstrual period and associated health and symptom tracking. Clue is designed so that, coupled with the guidance of a doctor, the app creates predictions and calendar reminders to best prepare for the different phases of your monthly cycle, which can improve overall health.

Similarly, Flo Period Tracker not only predicts when your next cycle will begin, it relies heavily on diet and exercise information you input to predict any type of changes in your cycle. It advises a woman when she will ovulate and which days fertility is at its peak. Women can log the symptoms of their periods and track them monthly, along with additional health and wellness facts, including sleep patterns. Like many of the other apps discussed in this chapter, Flo can also sync with other health apps or a Fitbit to more accurately gauge outside factors that could affect your period.

Nurx offers a digital application to enhance access to birth control. Like Lemonaid Health and Spruce, after a questionnaire is completed, a doctor prescribes a birth control pill that's most appropriate based on the patient's answers, current health, and budget. Pills are mailed directly to the patient's home and automatically renewed.

Although not all of these programs were necessarily designed exclusively for women, this step was included to showcase the positive impact that such programs and many other applications can play in your personal Health-Wealth plan. These applications and programs designed to assist women are all consistent with the overall 3P's formula to Health-Wealth, and each of these programs and applications would fit nicely into the 3P Plan of any woman seeking improved health and reduced wasteful healthcare spending.

HEALTH-WEALTH FOR BEHAVIORAL HEALTH, STRESS, AND ANXIETY

WITH THE RAPIDLY GROWING DEMAND for community-based behavioral health support and services, several national programs and applications have emerged that focus on reducing stress, more effectively managing anxiety, and focusing attention on behavioral and mental health. This rule highlights a few programs that can improve the Health-Wealth of individuals using tactics such as mindfulness, hypnotherapy, and relaxation tactics.

Perhaps the most well-known mainstream program is Headspace. Headspace is a web-based program that includes an application for mobile devices that teaches individuals how to effectively meditate and provides specific daily lessons in mindfulness. Headspace suggests that a commitment of just a few minutes a day and learning a few basic mindfulness skills is enough to make a significant difference in an individual's quality of life.

The Headspace approach is consistent with the integrative and functional medicine approaches discussed earlier. Natural remedies, including enhanced compassion, patience, and relaxation, are points of focus for this program. Although corporate programs are available, Headspace is an app that can be downloaded by anyone, and individuals can be participating within minutes and learning these new techniques.

Similarly, Calm.com is a natural, functional medicine approach to better manage mental health. The Calm website is headlined with the four words: meditate, sleep, wisdom, and music. The Daily Calm program is a daily lesson with more than a hundred guided meditations specific to managing anxiety, focus, stress, relationships, and other issues impacting mental health. Calm offers formal programs of seven days or three weeks for those who are just beginning the mindfulness process, all the way up to those who are advanced users.

As discussed previously, Clementine is a hypnotherapy application designed to help women feel confident. Clementine focuses on four key areas to relieve stress in women—sleep, confidence, de-stress, and mantras—and has proven beneficial for those who have utilized it. Clementine features a confidence-boost session and challenges you to describe what success looks like to you in your own words. Starting with visualization and a focus on imagery, the guide then progresses to goal-setting and forming an action plan. A constant theme is to shake off issues that arise and stay focused on your goals.

7 cups provides emotional support and counseling from trained active listeners who volunteer and are available 24/7 to connect via text chat. It also features three hundred free mindfulness exercises, videos, and mood-boosting activities. Like many of the other appli-

cations, 7 cups is free, and, of course, all callers and texters remain anonymous.

This list includes just a few of the resources available to those struggling with mental and behavioral issues. These applications and programs designed to assist with mental and behavioral health are all consistent with the overall 3P's formula to Health-Wealth: have a plan based on personalized and preventative medicine. Each of these programs and applications would fit nicely into the 3P plan of an individual who struggles with anxiety, stress, or behavioral-health issues. Not only will your stress and anxiety levels drop, but your health will improve, and you will eliminate wasteful healthcare spending along the way.

SOCKS WITH SANDALS

IN NOVEMBER 2014, I delivered my first-ever international keynote presentation. More than 300 executives from around the world, mostly from Central and South America, had come to hear me speak on how to control healthcare costs. I stood on the stage at the Trump International Hotel in Panama City, Panama, ready to reel off my opening joke, one that always makes a crowd laugh.

"I like to open my presentation with this PowerPoint slide for two reasons," I said with an anticipatory smile, preparing for the audience to respond to my next line with laughter, as was the norm. The slide listed a summary of my recent work history. "Not only does this opening slide show you my diverse professional background, but it also shows you that I can't keep a job for very long!" I said with a smile as I let out a loud chuckle.

Uh oh … no one else was laughing. A long, uncomfortable silence filled the room.

The crowd always loves that joke, I thought to myself. What went wrong? Was my delivery off? Did I butcher the punch line? I did a quick analysis in my head and realized where I miscalculated: English was a second language for the entire audience. The joke was lost in translation, and there was no turning back. I bombed it.

I rarely get nervous or sweat on stage, but within seconds, I felt perspiration overcome my body as the nerves kicked in.

"Quick," I thought, "get to the slide with the cute picture of my grandmother and tell the story of how I gave up private jets and celebrity sports marketing as a career to manage nursing homes. That always draws the crowd in."

"But wait, I have three or four other sure-fire jokes later in my presentation as well. Will those jokes bomb too? Will the crowd think it's funny in a few minutes when I emerge from behind the podium clad in Birkenstock sandals over red, polka-dot socks, so I can illustrate the contrasts between Gen Xers like me and millennials who think that socks with sandals are totally uncool?"

The nerves were running high. So, what did I do? I tried one more of my surefire one-liners. And it bombed as well.

I pivoted. I pivoted to material that was not likely to get lost in translation. I stuck to the facts on how to manage company expenses to keep healthcare from bankrupting a business. No more jokes, no more one-liners. Just the material. As the presentation evolved, with each of the remaining forty minutes, I saw the crowd become more engaged. Their posture improved, their facial expressions illustrated their interest, and I regained my confidence. I pivoted, and it worked. I was willing to try something new—avoid the humor and stick to the reason they came. They came to hear me speak because I am an expert sharing proven theories and experiences that can help them. I continued sharing simple tips that could save their families and businesses money by reducing wasteful healthcare spending.

That calculated pivot paid off for me. I finished strong and got several topical audience questions as I wrapped up my presentation. Individuals lined up to meet me when I was finished as well, and the event host advised me later that there was so much interest at the table outside the door that they sold out of copies of my most recent book, *Ex-Acute: A Former Hospital CEO Tells All on What's Wrong with American Healthcare.* A few weeks later, my audience feedback results came in very strong, and the event host subsequently hired me to present at several more events in coming years.

Since then I have presented in several other countries and always recall that my usual jokes and one-liners are a slippery slope. I still try my jokes in places like China and Germany, and audience responses can be hit and miss, but I won't be caught off guard again like I was in Panama!

While I hope I've entertained you along the way, like that Panamanian audience, you chose to read this book because you and your family deserve better from the healthcare you pay for. You deserve access to needed healthcare services at a reasonable, if not affordable price. You have the power and influence to pioneer this momentous turnabout for your family. And now you have the knowledge to begin the journey as well. This book represents your opportunity to pivot in the best interest of your family. The fact is that this decision and action plan are long overdue. But to date, no one has provided a road map on how to pivot—until now. You now have the roadmap, tools, and confidence to lead this change. Do you have the courage to lead this bold but necessary transformation?

Health-Wealth is your road map. And now that you have read the problem (Part I), identified that consumer-driven care and a

Health-Wealth culture are essential (Part II), and learned about tactics to consider (Part III), the next step is to prepare your 3P Plan to personal Health-Wealth by using the outline on the following pages. Another tool in preparing your #P Plan is to complete the online Health-Wealth Personal Loss Assessment. The assessment is a tool created to do a strengths, weaknesses, opportunities, threats (SWOT) analysis specific to healthcare spending. It was created to help identify where the biggest opportunity lies for you, someone who is ready to take back control of the main financial issue keeping your family from achieving your American dream. It's time to pro-actively manage your family's Health-Wealth just like you do with every other critical expense in your family budget.

Health-Wealth: the correlation between hyperinflating health-care costs and your family's declining net worth. Today your family starts bending the curve back to achieve both improved health and increased wealth. And it starts with you. You are the champion who leads the pivot … even if you, too, think that wearing socks with sandals is uncool and only for goofy old men!

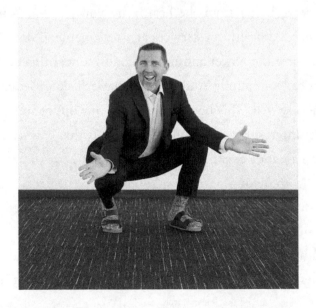

I started this book with the story of my family's Health-Wealth tipping point. And we pushed back. We took a chance. It was scary. We went without insurance for several months until I started a new job. Like us, other American families and businesses are reaching their Health-Wealth tipping point every day. And collectively, we've reached our Health-Wealth tipping point in America, and what's right is right. It's time to take a stand. I have been blessed with the tools and experience to lead the charge to Health-Wealth in America.

I've shown you why Health-Wealth is personal to me. What will it take to make it personal to you?

MY TOP FIVE GOALS TO ACHIEVE HEALTH-WEALTH

Goal #1: _____

How I intend to accomplish this:

_____

_____

Goal #2: _____

How I intend to accomplish this:

_____

_____

Goal #3: _____

How I intend to accomplish this:

_____

_____

Goal #4. _____

How I intend to accomplish this:

_____

_____

Goal #5: _____

How I intend to accomplish this:

_____

_____

Step #1

Enroll in an Alternative Insurance Model

Step #2

Engage in Integrative and Functional Medicine Approaches

Step #3

Full Genome Sequencing and DNA Testing

Step #4

Utilize Artificial Intelligence, Blockchain, and Machine Learning to Improve Your Health

Step #5

Utilize Telehealth and Remote Monitoring Services

Step #6

Participate in Local Medical Tourism

Step #7

Enroll in Disease-Specific Value Programs for Family Members with Chronic Diseases

Step #8

Convert to a Plan Offering Direct Primary Care

Step #9

Use Alternative Approaches to Buying Medication

Step #10

Health-Wealth for Women

Step #11

Health-Wealth for Behavioral Health, Stress, and Anxiety

A Partial Sampling of Questions
from the Online Assessment

1. I am answering as an:

   a. Individual

   b. Couple

   c. Family (Individual or couple with at least one child)

2. How many times a week do you (person completing assessment) exercise?

   a. Never

   b. 1-2

   c. 3 or more

3. Do you or anyone in your household have a chronic condition, chronic pain, or any other ongoing health issue?

   a. Yes

   b. No

   c. Unsure

4. Are you in a high deductible health plan at present?

   a. Yes

   b. No

   c. Not sure

5. Do you spend more than $100 monthly on medication for you or those in your household?

   a. Yes

   b. No

   c. Unsure

6. Is your health insurance provided by your (or spouses) company or do you contract on your own?

   a. Company

   b. On our own

   c. I am covered by Medicare, Medicaid, military (Tri-Care), or VA benefit

7. What is your households monthly share (cost) for your health insurance?

   a. Less than $500 per month

   b. $501 - $750 per month

   c. $751 - $1,000

   d. More than $1,001 per month

This is a sampling of just a few questions form the Personal Loss Assessment. Go online now to complete the full assessment and get a prompt email summarizing your savings opportunity!

Visit Health-Wealth.com and click on "Personal Loss Assessment" to complete and be eligible for preferred provider rates with all Health-Wealth Certified Partners.

CPSIA information can be obtained
at www.ICGtesting.com
Printed in the USA
BVHW041022230519
549097BV00008B/18/P

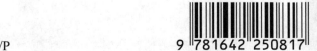